The U.S. Health Care Delivery System

Fundamental Facts, Definitions, and Statistics

D1560966

Kim M. Garber, Editor
American Hospital Association Resource Center

Health Forum, Inc.
An American Hospital Association Company
CHICAGO

press

AHA press and American Hospital Association are service marks of the American Hospital Association and are used under license by Health Forum, Inc.

Copyright © 2006 by Health Forum, Inc., an American Hospital Association company. All rights reserved. No part of this publication may be reproduced, stored in a retrieval system, or transmitted, in any form or by any means—electronic, mechanical, photocopying, recording, or otherwise—without the prior written permission of the publisher.

Printed in the United States of America—06/06

Cover design by Tim Kaage

ISBN 10: 1-55648-330-9   ISBN 13: 978-1-55648-330-1   Item Number: 196163

Discounts on bulk quantities of books published by Health Forum, Inc., are available to professional associations, special marketers, educators, trainers, and others. For details and discount information, contact Health Forum, Inc., One North Franklin, 28th Floor, Chicago, IL 60606-3421 (Phone: 1-800-242-2626).

Library of Congress Cataloging-in-Publication Data

The U.S. health care delivery system : fundamental facts, definitions, and statistics / Kim M. Garber, editor.
  p. cm.
 Includes bibliographical references and index.
 ISBN 1-55648-330-9 (softcover)
 1. Medical care—United States. 2. Medical care—United States—Forecasting. 3. Social medicine—United States. I. Garber, Kim M., 1953–. II. American Hospital Association. III. Title: Health system basics.
 RA445.U85 2006
 362.10973—dc22
              2006041182

Contents

List of Figures and Tables

Sara A. Beazley has worked in the American Hospital Association Resource Center since 1988 and is a senior information specialist, overseeing the custom information and data retrieval services provided by the resource center staff. Beazley indexed the hospital and health care administration journal literature under a cooperative arrangement with the National Library of Medicine to produce the Health Planning and Administration Database (HealthSTAR); she also oversaw the production of the *Hospital and Health Administration Index*. Prior to her employment at the American Hospital Association, Beazley spent six years at a Chicago law firm library, the last two as chief librarian. She has a master's degree in library science from the University of Chicago. She can be reached at sbeazley@aha.org.

Diana Culbertson is a senior information specialist with the American Hospital Association, where one of her key responsibilities is to provide information research on a wide range of health care topics. Culbertson was involved in the production of the former HealthSTAR database and the *Hospital and Health Administration Index*, collaboratively published by the American Hospital Association and the National Library of Medicine. She is active in the Special Libraries Association and serves on the editorial board of *Medicine on the Net*. Prior to her employment at the American Hospital Association, Culbertson worked for the Center for Business Knowledge at Ernst and Young and for several professional and trade associations. She has a master's degree in library science and has been credentialed as a senior member of the Academy of Health Information Professionals of the Medical Library Association. She can be reached at dculbertson@aha.org.

Kim M. Garber is an information specialist in the American Hospital Association Resource Center, where she is responsible for responding to a wide range of telephone and e-mail inquiries about health care–related issues. Garber has more than 25 years of experience as a health care librarian; in the past, she has worked for PricewaterhouseCoopers and the consulting firm of Herman Smith Associates, where she edited the *Library Bulletin* newsletter. She has a bachelor's degree in journalism and a master's degree in library science. She can be reached at kgarber@aha.org.

Jeanette M. Harlow is the director of the American Hospital Association Resource Center, where she not only manages the operation of the Resource Center but also provides information and research services to a wide range of clientele. Prior to her employment at the American Hospital Association, Harlow was the manager of the library of the Illinois Institute of Technology Research Institute. She was one of the developers of and instructors for *Health Care Administration Information Resources*, a Medical Library Association continuing-education course. She has a bachelor's degree in English and a master's degree in library science. She can be reached at jharlow@aha.org.

Rebecca J. Marthey is an information specialist in the American Hospital Association Resource Center, where she is responsible for managing the document delivery service. Prior to her employment at the American Hospital Association, Marthey was an information specialist with the Technical Information Service at Purdue University. She has also worked with a multi-type library network and has served as a school librarian in Indiana. She has a bachelor's degree in education and a master's degree in library science. She can be reached at rmarthey@aha.org.

Being a volunteer trustee of a hospital is not only a great honor; it is also an awesome responsibility. Trustees must remain true to the mission of the hospital and ensure that quality and safe services are provided to all patients, while adhering to numerous legal guidelines and maintaining the financial integrity of the institution.

Many trustees serve out of a sense of responsibility to their communities and often do not have extensive backgrounds in the health care arena. Trustees devote a great deal of time and energy to hospital and health care issues while juggling multiple responsibilities with their careers and families. The meeting agendas are usually packed with essential information about operations and administration that is needed to keep up with the constant changes in the very complex health care arena; therefore, little time is left for trustee education during the meetings. This reality makes it essential that hospital CEOs work with trustees to ensure that the trustees are able to access the information they need in order to fulfill their responsibilities.

The word *trustee* implies that trust is inherent in the position. Communities trust boards of trustees to properly oversee the management of the affairs of the hospitals in an ethical manner, while making sure that the values of all people in the community are represented in the decision-making process. Hospitals are rightly viewed as community assets, and some decisions that are made by boards of trustees can have serious consequences for the hospital as well as the community. This tremendous responsibility requires that trustees obtain a strong understanding of the health care field and be knowledgeable about current trends that will impact their decision making. Trustees must also utilize their understanding of the economics and demographics of their communities to address the health care needs of citizens in the communities they serve.

The delivery of health care in America is impacted by many factors. Some of the most significant changes are often made by legislators and regulators at the federal and state levels. Trustees must have a strong understanding of the impact of legislation on the governance and operation of hospitals. They should be knowledgeable enough to explain to lawmakers how legislation and regulations impact the hospitals they serve. Trustees must be strong advocates at all levels, help shape the public debate, and ultimately influence the development of regulations and policies. This is not possible unless the trustee has a good understanding of all facets of health care delivery.

In my role as a trustee, I have found that it is essential to become educated in order to fulfill my role as a trustee and health care advocate. Without health care education, it is impossible to carry out the legal responsibilities of a trustee or effectively represent the health care needs of the community that appointed me. The American Hospital Association, Health Forum, and the North Carolina Hospital Association have provided many opportunities for me to enhance my knowledge of the very complex health care industry. Through trustee seminars, conferences, and publications, in addition to participation on various committees and task forces, I continue to gain insight that will help me fulfill my responsibilities.

The U.S. Health Care Delivery System, written by members of the association's resource center, is an excellent way for all trustees to gain a basic understanding of the many factors that impact the delivery of health care in America. Organized by major topic—patient care, caregivers, facilities, funding, and government and oversight—the book provides both new and seasoned trustees with knowledge that is essential to fulfilling their legal, ethical, and moral duties. I challenge each board member and CEO to read and share this informative book in order to ensure that the future of hospitals in our nation is directed by informed and educated trustees.

Thomasine Kennedy
Trustee, Duplin General Hospital
Kenansville, North Carolina

North Carolina Trustee of the Year

Acknowledgments

We would like to thank Richard Hill, Sharon McDaniel, and Julie Melvin for their help in preparing and editing the manuscript.

To learn more about the information services available through the American Hospital Association Resource Center, please contact the resource center.

AHA Resource Center
American Hospital Association
One North Franklin
Chicago, IL 60606 USA
Phone: 312-422-2050
Fax: 312-422-4700
Email: rc@aha.org
Website: www.aha.org/resource/

The U.S. Health Care Delivery System

First, the patient, second the patient, third the patient, fourth the patient, fifth the patient, and then maybe comes science. We first do everything for the patient; science can wait, research can wait.[1]

(Dr. Bela Schick, 1877–1967)

Practicing in Vienna, and later in New York City, in the early twentieth century, eminent pediatrician Bela Schick was an accomplished scientist. He studied infectious diseases and established the Schick test to determine susceptibility to diphtheria. Yet, in his quote, "First the patient, second the patient, third the patient . . . ," Dr. Schick reminds us of the priorities of patient care. In these values, he echoes the teachings of Hippocrates, who wrote this advice to physicians in the fourth century B.C.E., "As to diseases, make a habit of two things—to help, or at least, to do no harm." Hippocrates identifies the central relationship in patient care as the interaction between the patient and the caregiver, with the focus on the patient.

Patient characteristics and some of the issues affecting caregivers will be explored in this chapter. A more detailed description of physicians, nurses, and other caregivers will be continued in chapter 2.

Patients

Despite the complexity of the health care system and of the challenges of running it, the practice of health care boils down to something simple to understand. It's all about the patients. Hospitals, doctors' offices, and all the other places where health care is delivered are full of highly trained professionals who take care of the sick and help the healthy stay well. As Dr. Will Mayo (1861–1939), one of the founders of the Mayo Clinic, said, "The best interest of the patient is the only interest to be considered." This chapter begins by describing the people of the United States, since we are all likely to be patients at some point in our lives.

Demographics

We live in a nation of nearly 300 million people that is growing by about 1 percent, or 3 million people, each year. Population growth is the result of both immigration and natural increase, defined as a greater number of births than deaths.

We have always been a nation of immigrants. In recent years, about 1 million legal immigrants and 300,000 undocumented immigrants have entered the country annually. Roughly one-third of legal immigrants come from elsewhere in North America, primarily from Mexico; another third come from Asia; and the rest arrive from other parts of the world. Today's immigrants are more likely than previous generations to want to retain their culture, customs, and language, portending even greater diversity in the future U.S. population.[2]

About 4 million babies are born in the United States each year. The annual number of births has varied little over the past few decades while the total population has increased. This translates to a drop in the birth rate—or number of live births per 1,000 population—from 24 in 1950 to 14 today. Likewise, the fertility rate—or number of live births to women of childbearing age—has decreased from 106 per 1,000 in 1950 to 65 per 1,000 today.[3]

Complementing the drop in the birth rate in the last half of the twentieth century has been an increase in longevity. Thanks to improvements in sanitation and medical care, people today can expect to live longer. A baby born today can expect to live to age 77, which is 30 years longer than the life expectancy of his great-grandfather born in 1900. Another mortality indicator, the age-adjusted death rate, has dropped from 14 per 1,000 population in 1950 to 9 per 1,000 as of the year 2000.[4]

Table 1–1. Total U.S. Population: Projections to 2050		
Year	Total	Change
2000	282,125,000	n/a
2010	308,936,000	10%
2020	335,805,000	9%
2030	363,584,000	8%
2040	391,946,000	8%
2050	419,854,000	7%

Source: U.S. Census Bureau, *U.S. Interim Projections by Age, Sex, Race, and Hispanic Origin* (March 18, 2004), http://www.census.gov/ipc/www/usinterimproj/ (accessed September 26, 2005).

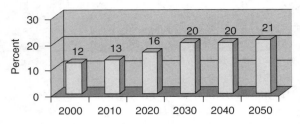

Figure 1–1. Percentage of population age 65 and over.

Source: U.S. Census Bureau, *U.S. Interim Projections by Age, Sex, Race, and Hispanic Origin* (March 18, 2004).

When will we reach 400 million?

The population of nearly 300 million Americans counted in the 2000 census will grow to 400 million by around the year 2040, as shown in table 1–1. Different racial and ethnic groups are projected to grow at widely differing rates over the next half century. The number of non-Hispanic whites will grow slowly while the Hispanic and Asian American populations will increase at a much higher rate. By 2050, nearly one-quarter of the population will be Hispanic.[5]

What happens when the Baby Boomers turn 65?

The aging of the American population has profound implications for the health care system. Baby Boomers will begin to reach retirement age in 2011 and will continue to increase the size of the senior population through 2029. In 2010, on the cusp of the Baby Boomer retirement trend, there will be an estimated 40 million seniors. Ten years later, the total will jump to 55 million and by 2030 will reach 71 million. Another way to describe the elderly population is as a percentage of the total population, as shown in figure 1–1. In 50 years, 1 in 5 Americans will be of retirement age, compared with about 1 in 10 today.[6]

How many people live in poverty?

About 37 million people, or nearly 13 percent of the U.S. population, live in poverty, according to 2004 statistics. The rate is higher for African Americans (25 percent), Hispanics (22 percent), women who are heads of households (28 percent), and noncitizens (22 percent). Thirteen million children (18 percent) live in poverty. Over the past 40 years, a positive trend has been the decreasing percentage of the elderly who live in poverty.

Sadly, however, the percentage of children living in poverty has been consistently higher than the percentage of adults since the mid-1970s.[7]

How many people have no health insurance?

A snapshot of the Americans without health insurance bears some resemblance to those living in poverty. Just under 46 million people, or 16 percent of the population, were without health insurance in 2004. As shown in figure 1–2, lack of health insurance tends to be a problem of young adults and children. Over one-quarter of young adults (under age 35) and 11 percent of children have no health insurance. About one-quarter of low-income people, one-fifth of blacks, and nearly one-third of Hispanics are uninsured. Nearly one-half of noncitizens have no coverage. In contrast, less than 1 percent of senior citizens are uninsured. Since the late 1980s, both the total number and the percentage of uninsured Americans have shown an overall upward trend.[8]

Are we patients or are we consumers?

Over the past few decades, there has been a rise in consumerism in health care. People today are more likely to evaluate care options, comparing cost, quality, and convenience factors among providers. People are more likely to initiate their own diagnostic testing and elective surgery. As the influential Baby Boom generation ages, this trend is likely to continue.[9]

Health Status

How have disease patterns changed?

Modern medicine and improved public sanitation have transformed the pattern of illness in the United States. Communicable diseases such as measles, polio, and diphtheria that once infected hundreds of thousands have been controlled through routine childhood vaccination. Deaths

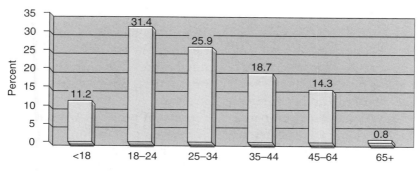

Figure 1–2. Uninsured by age group: United States, 2004.

Source: U.S. Census Bureau, "Income, Poverty, and Health Insurance Coverage in the United States, 2004," *Current Population Reports* P60, no. 229 (August 2005): 18, http://www.census.gov/prod/2005pubs/p60-229.pdf (accessed November 1, 2005).

caused by acute illnesses, such as influenza and pneumonia, dropped significantly during the last half of the twentieth century. But because people are living longer, they are more likely to suffer chronic diseases. Additionally, AIDS illustrates the potential for the emergence of new disease conditions.[10]

What are the leading causes of illness and death?

The top three causes of death have remained unchanged over the past 20 years: heart disease, cancer, and cerebrovascular disease. Rounding out the top five causes of death today are chronic lower respiratory diseases and unintentional injuries. According to the American Heart Association, 70 million Americans, or roughly a quarter of the population, have some form of cardiovascular disease. Each year about 865,000 people suffer a heart attack and 700,000 have a stroke. The total direct and indirect cost to the nation associated with cardiovascular disease has been estimated at $394 billion for 2005. The aging of the population, along with the growing numbers of overweight people and those with diabetes, are expected to fuel continued growth in the incidence of cardiovascular disease.[11]

In 2005 over a million Americans learned that they have cancer. Prostate cancer and breast cancer are by far the most common types, followed by lung and colon cancer. Cancer cost the nation about $190 billion in direct and indirect costs in 2004, according to the National Institutes of Health.[12]

Do we feel well?

Roughly 1 in 10 Americans rate themselves as having only "fair" or "poor" health. Twelve percent

report that they are limited in their activities due to a chronic condition, most often arthritis or another musculoskeletal problem. Not surprisingly, both the perception of poor health and the limitation on activities increase with age. About one-third of seniors aged 75 or older describe their health as less than good, and nearly half say that they have activity limitations. Minorities and low-income people are more likely to report poor health status.[13]

Are we taking good care of ourselves?

Early prenatal care is an important first step in protecting an individual's lifetime health. Over the past 30 years, the percentage of women who have sought prenatal care during the first trimester of pregnancy has been steadily increasing. Today, over 80 percent receive this care. An encouraging related trend has been a decrease in the percentage of women who smoke during pregnancy. Despite these positive indicators, however, the percentage of low-birthweight newborns has remained constant over the past 30 years, at about 7 to 8 percent of live births. Over the same period, the percentage of very-low-birthweight babies has also remained steady, at about 1 percent of births. Despite the lack of improvement in these birthweight indicators, the infant mortality rate has been decreasing since the mid-1980s.[14]

Vaccination rates for toddlers have shown an encouraging trend in recent years. About 80 to 90 percent of young children are receiving vaccinations against the major preventable contagious diseases. As is true with other health care access issues, children living in poverty are somewhat less likely to be vaccinated, but the rates are still fairly uniform across income groups.[15]

Smoking is the number one cause of preventable disease in the United States. The good news is that cigarette smoking is less prevalent than it was 30 years ago. About one-quarter of adults report themselves as current cigarette smokers, compared with 42 percent in 1965. But young adults continue to have a comparatively high rate of smokers. In a 2002 survey, 45 percent of young adults aged 18 to 25 reported the use of some type of tobacco product within the past 12 months. Generally speaking, people with higher levels of education are less likely to smoke.[16]

Half of all teens and adults drink alcohol, and 7 percent are heavy drinkers. Young adults, aged 18 to 34, are the most likely to drink, while teens and young adults are the most likely to use illicit drugs. Eight percent of all teens and adults use drugs.[17]

Two-thirds of high school students take part in the recommended amount of physical activity. However, only about one-third of adults report achieving a medium level of exercise. Inactivity tends to increase with age, and women are generally more likely to be inactive than men.[18]

How serious a problem is obesity?

Lack of exercise and poor eating habits are among the leading causes of a significant health problem facing American society today: obesity. Even more sobering than the growth in the overall number of overweight Americans is the fact that so many adolescents and children are affected and face a lifelong battle with weight control. Poor eating habits and lack of physical activity have led to a dramatic increase in the number of people who are overweight over the past 40 years. Currently, two-thirds of the adult population (ages 20–74 years) are classified as overweight, and nearly one-third as obese. Black women are particularly at risk: fully half meet the clinical requirements for obesity. An estimated 9 million children and youth have a weight problem. Medical care for obesity and related conditions reportedly represented 27 percent of the growth in health care spending between 1987 and 2001. The total cost to the nation of medical care associated with obesity is estimated at $93 billion each year.[19]

Is there a diabetes epidemic?

Diabetes, one of the many health problems commonly associated with obesity, has been called a worldwide epidemic. An estimated 18 million people in the United States have the disease, but 5 million of these have not been diagnosed. This represents 6 percent of the population. Because the incidence of diabetes increases with age, it will become an even more significant problem with the aging of the American population. Projections indicate a potential 225 percent increase in the prevalence of diabetes in the next 50 years.[20]

Is life becoming overly medicalized?

On the subject of disease patterns and health care habits, it is worth noting that some physicians are becoming concerned about the growing medicalization of life in the industrialized world. There is a growing perception that problems once regarded as a normal part of life or aging, such as menopause, are now considered medical conditions to be treated. This perception leads to increased health care utilization and a greater consumption of drugs, with the concomitant possibility of side effects.[21]

Health Care Overview

Most Americans have a doctor's office or other provider that they consider their usual source of health care. In 2003 only 14 percent of adults reported that they had no usual place of care, according to the National Health Interview Survey. Not surprisingly, the uninsured were far more likely (44 percent) to report having no usual place of care. For most people who responded to this survey, the doctor's office or HMO is the provider they turn to first. About 16 percent mentioned clinics, and 3 percent rely on the hospital emergency room or outpatient department.[22]

Health Services Utilization Overview

What drives health services utilization?

Key drivers of health services utilization include access to care, demographics, new medical technology and drugs, and the emergence of new disease patterns. Access to care is determined by the availability of health insurance coverage as well as the physical location of health care resources. As noted previously, changes in the demographics of the American people over the next decades will have a significant impact on the demand for health care services. In addition, the rapid dissemination of information about the development of new technologies, procedures, and pharmaceuticals is likely to ramp up demand among health care consumers. The emergence of entirely new diseases and conditions, such as AIDS or bioterrorism agents, or changes in chronic disease patterns will also affect utilization. In a 2005 overview of the not-for-profit health care sector, Moody's Investors Service projects that the aging of the population combined with medical technology innovations will result in long-term growth in hospital utilization.[23]

Is health care a right or a privilege?

Presidential candidate John Kerry stated in his acceptance speech before the 2004 Democratic National Convention, "And when I am president, we will stop being the only advanced nation in the world which fails to understand that health care is not a privilege for the wealthy, and the connected and the elected; it is a right for all Americans." In this sentiment, Kerry echoed a campaign promise of Bill Clinton some 10 years earlier. The issue of whether to reform the health care system to guarantee universal access to at least a basic set of health care services remains unresolved. One commentator has pointed out that in the United States, only prisoners and patients needing emergency care have been granted a right to health services, while another observer notes that consumers in a free market economy are generally expected to provide for themselves.[24]

How often do we visit doctors?

About 1 in 5 adults did not visit a doctor at all in 2003, but the average person makes three office visits per year. This amounts to just over 900 million physician office visits a year, as shown in table 1–2. For adults, the likelihood of visiting the doctor increases with age. Young adults see a physician about twice a year, on average, while senior citizens make six to seven doctor visits annually. Therefore, as the U.S. population as a whole ages, the demand for physician office care is likely to increase.[25]

Roughly two-thirds of physician office visits are paid for through private insurance, with Medicaid (or the State Children's Health Insurance Program) the second most common payor. The usual outcome of a physician office visit is to schedule a return appointment. Less than 1 percent of office visits result in admission to the hospital.[26]

Table 1–2. Number of Physician Office Visits per Year		
Year	Total Office Visits	Visits/Person
1993	717,191,000	2.8
1994	681,457,000	2.6
1995	697,082,000	2.7
1996	734,493,000	2.8
1997	787,372,000	3.0
1998	829,280,000	3.1
1999	756,734,000	2.8
2000	823,542,000	3.0
2001	880,487,000	3.1
2002	889,980,000	3.1
2003	906,023,000	3.2

Source: U.S. Department of Health and Human Services, "National Ambulatory Medical Care Survey: 2003 Summary," *Advance Data* 365 (October 4, 2005), and earlier editions, http://www.cdc.gov/nchs/data/ad/ad365.pdf (accessed November 1, 2005).

How often do we use alternative therapies?

The use of complementary and alternative medicine (CAM), such as acupuncture or chiropractic, has grown during the past decade. According to a 2002 national survey, some 124 million people, or two-thirds of adults in the United States, reported using some type of CAM during the previous year. Included among the list of CAM therapies was prayer, which was by far the most commonly cited therapy by survey respondents. Other leading CAM choices were herbal medicine, chiropractic, and deep breathing exercises.[27]

Do people use the emergency room inappropriately?

In 2002 the American Hospital Association (AHA) conducted a national survey that found approximately 80 percent of urban hospital emergency departments to be "at capacity" or "over capacity." In addition, over half of these urban providers reported that they had spent time on ambulance diversion status, which means that the hospital emergency department (ED) was too full to accept any patients or certain types of patients coming in by ambulance for a period of time. In a more recent detailed follow-up of the ED situation in four cities, the AHA again found that over half of hospital EDs reported being "at capacity" or "over capacity." Among the factors contributing to crowded emergency departments are local population growth, inadequate availability of physicians, and lack of community resources to care for Medicaid patients.[28]

Data on the nature of visits to emergency departments are collected by the National Center for Health Statistics. In 2003, 13 percent of visits to U.S. emergency departments were classified as nonurgent and another 20 percent as semiurgent. Emergency department visits were more likely to be nonurgent for children than for any other age group. Nearly half of patient visits that were identified by expected source of payment as "no charge" were nonurgent. Medicaid patients' visits were more likely to be nonurgent than Medicare patients' visits.[29]

Selected Trends in Medical Practice

Is there still a trend toward substituting ambulatory for inpatient care?

Health care today is delivered predominantly in ambulatory settings. The most common ambulatory care setting is the physician's office, with hospital outpatient clinics and emergency departments each accounting for about 10 percent of all ambulatory care visits.[30] One of the most striking trends in health care over the past half century has been the development of ambulatory alternatives to care that previously would have been offered only in the inpatient setting.

An interesting example of this substitution of ambulatory for inpatient care is the explosion in ambulatory surgery since the 1970s. As shown in table 1–3, the percentage of outpatient surgery at U.S. registered community hospitals has grown steadily until reaching a plateau in this decade. Today, two-thirds of all surgical procedures performed at U.S. registered community hospitals are done on an outpatient basis. Moreover, the total number of outpatient surgical procedures is even greater than shown in table 1–3, which does not include procedures performed in independently owned, freestanding outpatient surgery centers or in physician's offices.

Are minimally invasive procedures the future of surgery?

Many Americans have undergone open-heart surgery, hip replacement surgery, or other major surgical procedures involving long incisions and lengthy recovery times. Less traumatic options are becoming available for an increasing number of patients. Cardiac surgeons have developed new bypass surgery techniques that sound like science fiction: off-pump procedures done on the beating heart, minimally invasive procedures done through small keyhole incisions, and robotic procedures in which the surgeon does not directly touch the patient at all. In 2000 a surgical team in Pittsburgh pioneered a minimally invasive bypass procedure on an awake patient treated with local anesthesia only.[31]

Cardiac surgeons are not the only specialists working with minimally invasive techniques. At Baylor University Medical Center surgeons have developed a laparoscopic version of the gastric bypass for obese patients. It was estimated that in 2004, 75 percent of the Baylor patients having this procedure would be outpatients, leaving the hospital within 23 hours. This is a significant improvement over the complex open gastric bypass procedure, which requires a several-day post-op stay. The soaring numbers of overweight Americans make developments in the bariatric surgery field important to monitor.[32]

Orthopedics is another specialty facing change with the development of minimally invasive procedures. Minimally invasive techniques for both total hip and total knee replacement are gaining popularity with patients, although some physicians caution that long-term outcome studies are needed. In Chicago and in Pittsburgh, surgeons have pushed the envelope even further and pioneered not only minimally invasive but also outpatient total hip and total knee replacements.[33]

Table 1–3. Growth in Outpatient Surgery, 1980–2004: All U.S. Registered Community Hospitals

| Year | Number of Surgeries | | | Percent | |
	Inpatient	Outpatient	Total	Inpatient	Outpatient
2004	10,050,346	17,351,490	27,401,836	37	63
2000	9,729,336	16,383,374	26,112,710	37	63
1995	9,700,613	13,462,304	23,162,917	42	58
1990	10,844,916	11,069,952	21,914,868	49	51
1980	15,714,062	3,053,604	18,767,666	84	16

Source: American Hospital Association, *AHA Hospital Statistics*, 2006 ed. (Chicago: Health Forum, 2006): 11, and earlier editions.

What's happening with robotics?

Leading hospitals are experimenting with robotics in a variety of clinical applications. In surgery, the use of robots continues the evolution of minimally invasive procedures by allowing the physician to operate from a remote console without touching the patient. Robotic procedures have been developed for gallbladder removal, coronary bypass, and prostate cancer surgery. In March 2005 robotic surgery was performed at the University of Iowa Hospital on a 6-pound newborn with a life-threatening hole in her diaphragm.[34]

Another new development that has proved popular with patients and their families has been a teleconferencing robot that makes rounds on patient care units. The robot has a television screen broadcasting a live video image of the physician's face, and it drives around the hospital by remote control to allow the physician to talk with patients. The UCLA Medical Center is using this approach to monitor patients in the neurosurgery intensive care unit.[35]

In other applications, Cincinnati Children's Hospital Medical Center is among the pioneers using a robotic device to mix intravenous medications. The robot, also capable of preparing syringes, is particularly useful in a pediatric hospital, where medication doses must be calibrated according to the patient's weight. The hospital hopes that the new system will help achieve the goal of eliminating medication errors.[36]

How will genomics change medical care?

In the opening years of this century, the 20,000 to 25,000 key genes in the human body were identified and sequenced. This remarkable scientific achievement has been followed by an even more challenging quest—proteomics, which seeks to identify all the proteins in the body and how they work.[37]

The development of personalized, or targeted, medicine, in which diagnosis and treatment are specifically tailored to a specific disease or group of patients, is expected from genomic and proteomic research. Farther in the future may be the advent of individualized medicine, customized to the individual based on his or her genetic characteristics. A major new initiative targeting a specific disease is the proposed Human Cancer Genome Project, which is expected to cost at least $1 billion over nine years. Another promising area is a public-private joint venture to study the genetic causes of diabetes.[38]

The development of new therapies based on genomics and proteomics research has interesting implications for hospitals. As imaging departments have done in the recent past, hospital clinical laboratories in the future may develop beyond their purely diagnostic function to include an interventional component. Hospitals may find an opportunity to promote an interventional lab, working in close collaboration with the hospital pharmacy, as a leading-edge service. Hospitals are also seeking opportunities to collaborate on genomics applications research, such as the program at the new Phoenix Biomedical Center.[39]

What is the role of early diagnosis?

At first glance, the value of early diagnosis seems obvious. Who would contest the idea of catching a disease early so that treatment can be initiated promptly? Cancer provides a well-known example. The American Cancer Society advocates early detection of a variety of types of cancer through the screening of individuals who do not have symptoms. This screening has become a routine part of normal primary care in the United States—from Pap tests to periodic mammograms to prostate exams.[40]

Mass screening of asymptomatic individuals does present issues, however. One of these is overdiagnosis, or the identification of disease conditions that would not otherwise have been detected in the patient's lifetime. A recent study of prostate cancer screening found a "remarkably high" probability of overdiagnosis. Another aspect of overdiagnosis has been observed with women who have mammograms showing small, suspicious abnormalities and who typically opt for treatment rather than adopt a watchful waiting approach. Other issues with mass screening pertain to the cost-effectiveness of screening large numbers of people, the degree of invasiveness of the test, and whether effective treatment is available.[41]

Does health care still lag other industries in investing in IT?

In 2006 the health care industry will spend nearly $31 billion on health information technology, compared with $19 billion in 2000, according to industry analysts Sheldon I. Dorenfest & Associates. This robust IT market growth is led by purchases of picture archiving and communications systems (PACS) and computerized physician order entry

(CPOE) systems, Dorenfest reports. The commonly held belief that health care organizations invest much less in IT than do other industries has been challenged by two studies. Both compared health care IT expenditures as a percentage of revenue with a corresponding metric for the banking and financial services industry. In 2001 banking and financial services spent about 5 to 6 percent of revenues on IT, compared with 3 to 4 percent for health care organizations. More current data from a *Modern Healthcare*–PricewaterhouseCoopers annual survey of hospital executives indicate that the typical health care organization allocates 2.5 percent of the operating budget to information technology.[42]

Senior hospital executives responding to the *Modern Healthcare* 2005 survey indicated their primary near-term IT priority to be the electronic health record (EHR). A key impetus in the increased interest in the EHR was the 2004 pledge by President George W. Bush to establish an interoperable system of health records within a decade and the appointment of the first national coordinator of health information technology to oversee the process. The total national cost of introducing this system has been estimated at $276 to $320 billion over 10 years. The cost to a medium-sized hospital has been estimated at $2.7 million initially and then $250,000 per year. Annual savings achievable with a fully operating system have been estimated at $77.8 billion nationally and $1.3 million for that medium-sized hospital. Some industry observers believe that the challenges of building such a national infrastructure are comparable to those of putting a man on the moon, and that the project is likely to require several decades to complete. However, the potential benefits associated with the EHR in terms of patient care and medical research are compelling.[43]

What is technology's impact on patient care, safety, and longevity?
Advances in technology have had a profound impact on the delivery of patient care, particularly in the shift from inpatient to outpatient settings and in the development of ever more finely honed and less invasive diagnostic and therapeutic techniques. Among the futuristic inventions with the potential to improve patient safety is a microchip permanently implanted below the skin that, when scanned, provides immediate access to the patient's medical records or that can act as a sensor to monitor the

condition of chronic disease patients. An innovation currently being deployed in hospitals across the country is the eICU, in which monitoring of ICU patients is centralized in an off-site location, staffed by physician specialists and nurses. This system is expected to be in widespread use by 2010, according to a *Futurescan* survey of health care leaders.[44]

References

1. Maurice B. Strauss, ed., *Familiar Medical Quotations* (Boston, MA: Little, Brown and Company, 1968), 374.
2. U.S. Census Bureau, *Statistical Abstract of the United States 2003* (Washington, DC: Government Printing Office, 2003), http://www.census.gov/prod/2004pubs/03statab/pop.pdf (accessed April 28, 2005); U.S. Department of Homeland Security, *2002 Yearbook of Immigration Statistics* (Washington, DC: Government Printing Office, 2003), uscis.gov/graphics/shared/aboutus/ statistics/Yearbook2002.pdf (accessed April 28, 2005); Noah Rubin Brier, David Myron, and Christopher Reynolds, "Foresight Is 20/20," *American Demographics* 26, no. 6 (July/August 2004): 32–39; William H. Frey, "Zooming In on Diversity," *American Demographics* 26, no. 6 (July/August 2004): 27–31.
3. U.S. Department of Health and Human Services, *Health, United States, 2004* (Hyattsville, MD: National Center for Health Statistics, 2004), http://www.cdc.gov/nchs/data/hus/hus04trend.pdf#topic (accessed April 28, 2005); U.S. Census Bureau, "Fertility of American Women: June 2002," *Current Population Reports* P20, no. 548 (October 2003), http://www.census.gov/prod/2003pubs/p20-548.pdf (accessed April 28, 2005).
4. Ibid., 147.
5. U.S. Census Bureau, *U.S. Interim Projections by Age, Sex, Race, and Hispanic Origin* (March 18, 2004), www.census.gov/ipc/www/usinterimproj/ (accessed April 28, 2005).
6. Ibid.
7. U.S. Census Bureau, "Income, Poverty, and Health Insurance Coverage in the United States: 2004," *Current Population Reports* P60, no. 229 (August 2005), http://www.census.gov/prod/2005pubs/p60-229.pdf (accessed November 1, 2005).
8. Ibid.
9. Society for Healthcare Strategy and Market Development, *Futurescan: Healthcare Trends and Implications 2004–2008* (Chicago: Society for Healthcare Strategy and Market Development, 2004).
10. *Health, United States, 2004:* 146, 207; U.S. Centers for Disease Control, "Notice to Readers: Final 2003 Reports of Notifiable Diseases," *MMWR* 53, no. 30 (August 5, 2004): 687–696, http://www.cdc.gov/mmwr/preview/mmwrhtml/mm5330a6.htm (accessed April 28, 2005).

11. *Health, United States, 2004:* 154; American Heart Association, *Heart Disease and Stroke Statistics: 2005 Update* (Dallas, TX: American Heart Association, 2005), http://www.americanheart.org/downloadable/heart/1105390918119HDSStats2005Update.pdf (accessed April 28, 2005).

12. American Cancer Society, *Cancer Facts & Figures 2005* (Atlanta, GA: American Cancer Society, 2005), http://www.cancer.org/downloads/STT/CAFF2005f4PWSecured.pdf (accessed April 28, 2005).

13. *Health, United States, 2004:* 214–218.

14. Ibid.: 113–115, 120–125, 131–132.

15. Ibid.: 250–251.

16. Ibid.: 223–229.

17. Ibid.: 228, 235–237.

18. U.S. Department of Health and Human Services, *Health, United States, 2003* (Hyattsville, MD: National Center for Health Statistics, 2003): 72, http://www.cdc.gov/nchs/data/hus/hus03.pdf (accessed April 28, 2005).

19. Kenneth E. Thorpe, Curtis S. Florence, David H. Howard, et al., "The Impact of Obesity on Rising Medical Spending," *Health Affairs Web Exclusive* (October 20, 2004), http://content.healthaffairs.org/cgi/content/abstract/hlthaff.w4.480v1 (accessed March 24, 2005); Robert M. Kessler and Bettina Eckstein, "Obesity: Health Insurance Plans Respond to a Public Health Challenge," *AHIP Coverage* 46, no. 2 (March–April 2005): 38–40, 42.

20. American Diabetes Association, *National Diabetes Fact Sheet* (2002), https://www.diabetes.org/diabetes-statistics/national-diabetes-fact-sheet.jsp (accessed April 28, 2005); Michael M. Englegau, Linda S. Geiss, Jinan B. Saaddine, et al., "The Evolving Diabetes Burden in the United States," *Annals of Internal Medicine* 140, no. 11 (June 2004): 945–949.

21. Victoria S. Elliott, "Are We All Sick? Doctors Debate 'Medicalization' of Life," *American Medical News* (September 20, 2004).

22. U.S. Department of Health and Human Services, "Summary of Health Statistics for U.S. Adults: National Health Interview Survey, 2003," *Vital and Health Statistics* 10, no. 225 (July 2005), http://www.cdc.gov/nchs/data/series/sr_10/sr10_225.pdf (accessed November 1, 2005).

23. Moody's Investors Service, *Not-For-Profit Healthcare Sector: 2005 Industry Outlook* (January 2005).

24. "Text of John Kerry's Acceptance Speech at the Democratic National Convention," *Washington Post* (July 29, 2004), http://www.washingtonpost.com/wp-dyn/articles/A25678-2004Jul29.html (accessed April 28, 2005); Michael Wines and Robert Pear, "President Finds Benefits in Defeat on Health Care," *New York Times* (July 29, 1996); Howard Haft, "Is Health Care a Right or a Privilege?"

Physician Executive 29, no.1 (January–February 2003): 26–29; Phoebe Lindsey Barton, *Understanding the U.S. Health Services System*, 2nd ed. (Chicago: Health Administration Press, 2003): 45.

25. "Summary of Health Statistics for U.S. Adults"; U.S. Department of Health and Human Services, "National Ambulatory Medical Care Survey: 2003 Summary," *Advance Data* 365 (October 5, 2005), http://www.cdc.gov/nchs/data/ad/ad365.pdf (accessed November 1, 2005).

26. "National Ambulatory Medical Care Survey."

27. U.S. Department of Health and Human Services, "Complementary and Alternative Medicine Use Among Adults: United States, 2002," *Advance Data* 343 (May 27, 2004), http://www.cdc.gov/nchs/data/ad/ad343.pdf (accessed April 28, 2005).

28. Lewin Group, *Hospital Capacity and Emergency Department Diversion: Four Community Case Studies, AHA Survey Reports* (Chicago: American Hospital Association, April 2004), http://www.ahapolicyforum.org/ahapolicyforum/resources/content/EDDiversionSurvey040421.ppt (accessed April 28, 2005).

29. U.S. Department of Health and Human Services, "National Hospital Ambulatory Medical Care Survey: 2003 Emergency Department Summary," *Advance Data* 358 (May 26, 2005), http://www.cdc.gov/nchs/data/ad/ad358.pdf (accessed November 1, 2005).

30. Ibid.; U.S. Department of Health and Human Services, "National Hospital Ambulatory Medical Care Survey: 2002 Outpatient Department Summary," *Advance Data* 345 (June 24, 2004), http://www.cdc.gov/nchs/data/ad/ad345.pdf (accessed May 13, 2005).

31. University of Pittsburgh Medical Center, "Awake, Patient Undergoes Heart Bypass Surgery" (Press Release, July 5, 2000), http://newsbureau.upmc.com/pdf/FirstMidcab.pdf (accessed May 13, 2005); University of Maryland Medicine, *Minimally Invasive Heart Surgery* (May 17, 2002), http://www.umm.edu/ency/article/007012.htm (accessed May 13, 2005).

32. Todd McCarty, "Succeeding at Outpatient Gastric Bypass Surgery," *Outpatient Surgery Magazine* 5, no. 9 (September 2004), http://www.outpatientsurgery.net/2004/os09/succeeding_outpatient_gastric_bypass.php (accessed May 13, 2005).

33. Alicia Ault, "Less Invasive Hip & Knee Surgery Debated," *WebMD Medical News* (March 12, 2004), http://my.webmd.com/content/Article/83/97882.htm (accessed May 13, 2005); Rush University Medical Center, "Rush University Medical Center First to Perform Minimally Invasive Total Knee Replacement Surgery as Outpatient" (Press Release, February 6, 2004), http://www.rush.edu/webapps/MEDREL/servlet/NewsRelease?id=535 (accessed May 13,

2005); Sid Kirchheimer, "Get a New Hip, Walk Home That Day," *WebMD Medical News* (November 13, 2003), http://my.webmd.com/content/article/77/90340.htm (accessed May 13, 2005).

34. Cinda Becker, "Look, No Hands," *Modern Healthcare* 31, no. 18 (April 30, 2001): 36ff; Jen Waters, "A Revolution in Heart Surgery," *Washington Times* (February 8, 2005): B1; Todd Dvorak, "Infant Who Became the Smallest to Undergo Robotic Surgery Is Recovering," *Associated Press* (March 14, 2005), http://www.cp.org/premium/online/commercial/health/050314/x031416A.html (accessed May 13, 2005).

35. UCLA Medical Center, "UCLA Medical Center Becomes World's First Hospital to Introduce Remote Presence Robots in ICU" (March 9, 2005), http://www.newsroom.ucla.edu/page.asp?RelNum=5966 (accessed May 13, 2005); Arlene Weintraub, "Meet Mr. Rounder," *Business Week* (March 28, 2005), http://www.businessweek.com/magazine/content/05_13/b3926011_mz001.htm (accessed May 13, 2005).

36. Matt Leingang, "Rx Robot Does All Except Give Shot," *Cincinnati Enquirer* (January 4, 2005): 1, http://news.enquirer.com/apps/pbcs.dll/article?AID=/20050104/NEWS01/501040378 (accessed May 13, 2005).

37. International Human Genome Sequencing Consortium, "Finishing the Euchromatic Sequence of the Human Genome," *Nature* 431 (October 21, 2004): 931–945, http://www.nature.com/cgi-taf/DynaPage.taf?file=/nature/journal/v431/n7011/full/nature03001_fs.html&content_filetype=PDF (accessed May 13, 2005); Stanley Fields, "Proteomics in Genomeland," *Science* 291, no. 5507 (February 16, 2001): 1221–1224, http://www.sciencemag.org/cgi/content/full/291/5507/1221 (accessed May 13, 2005).

38. Andrew Pollak, "Huge Genome Project Is Proposed to Fight Cancer," *New York Times* (March 28, 2005): A1; Massachusetts Institute of Technology, "Broad, Novartis Announce Diabetes Initiative" (Press Release, October 28, 2004), http://web.mit.edu/newsoffice/2004/diabetes2.html (accessed May 13, 2005).

39. Jeff Goldsmith, "Technology and the Boundaries of the Hospital: Three Emerging Technologies," *Health Affairs* 23, no. 6 (November/December 2004): 149–156, http://content.healthaffairs.org/cgi/reprint/23/6/149 (accessed May 13, 2005); Angela Gonzales, "New TGen Facility Fills to Occupancy, Begins Research," *Business Journal of Phoenix* (February 4, 2005), http://phoenix.bizjournals.com/phoenix/stories/2005/02/07/story2.html?t=printable (accessed May 13, 2005).

40. American Cancer Society, "Early Detection" (December 2002), http://www.cancer.org/docroot/PED/content/PED_2_3X_Early_Detection.asp?sitearea=PED&viewmode=print& (accessed May 13, 2005).

41. Ori Davidov, "Overdiagnosis in Early Detection Programs," *Biostatistics* 5, no. 4 (2004): 603–613, http://biostatistics.oupjournals.org/cgi/content/abstract/5/4/603 (accessed May 13, 2005); Rita Rubin, "Breast Cancer Study Cites 'Overdiagnosis,'" *USA Today* (March 8, 2001), http://www.usatoday.com/news/health/2001-03-08-breast-cancer.htm (accessed May 13, 2005); R.M. Genta, "Screening for Gastric Cancer: Does It Make Sense?" *Alimentary Pharmacology & Therapeutics* 20, suppl. 2 (July 2004): 42–47, http://www.ncbi.nlm.nih.gov/entrez/query.fcgi?cmd=Retrieve&db=pubmed&dopt=Abstract&list_uids=15335412 (accessed May 13, 2005).

42. Sheldon I. Dorenfest & Associates, "Healthcare Information Technology Spending Is Growing Rapidly" (Press Release, February 2004), http://www.dorenfest.com/pressrelease_Feb2004.pdf (accessed May 13, 2005); Chris Parton and John P. Glaser, "Myths about IT spending," *Healthcare Informatics* 19, no. 7 (July 2002): 39–40, http://www.healthcare-informatics.com/issues/2002/07_02/myths.htm (accessed May 13, 2005); John Morrissey, "This Time They Really Mean It," *Modern Healthcare* 35, no. 7 (February 14, 2005): 42–50.

43. Morrissey, 42–50; Howard Larkin, "Uncle Sam Wants Your EHR," *Hospitals & Health Networks* 79, no. 2 (February 2005): 38ff, http://www.hhnmag.com/hhnmag/hospitalconnect/search/article.jsp?dcrpath=HHNMAG/PubsNewsArticle/data/0502HHN_FEA_CoverStory&domain=HHNMAG (accessed May 13, 2005).

44. Christopher Gearon, "IT's Inside You," *Hospitals & Health Networks* 79, no. 2 (February 2005): 22, http://www.hhnmag.com/hhnmag/hospitalconnect/search/article.jsp?dcrpath=HHNMAG/PubsNewsArticle/data/0502HHN_InBox_Technology&domain=HHNMAG (accessed May 13, 2005); Kevin Featherly, "Emerging Technologies," *Healthcare Informatics* 22, no. 1 (January 2005): 25ff, http://www.healthcare-informatics.com/issues/2005/01_05/cover.htm (accessed May 13, 2005); *Futurescan*, 18.

Health care is not just another service industry. Its fundamental nature is characterized by people taking care of other people in times of need and stress. Patients are ill, families are worried, and the ultimate outcome may be uncertain. Stable, trusting relationships between a patient and the people providing care can be critical to healing or managing an illness. The people who deliver care are the health system's most important resource.

(Institute of Medicine, *Crossing the Quality Chasm*, 2001)

Behind every medical examination, laboratory test, drug prescription, patient meal, or change of bed linen, there stands a person, whether it be a physician, a registered nurse, a laboratory technician, a pharmacist, or a member of the hospital's food service or housekeeping staff. This chapter provides an overview of the vast pool of human resources dedicated to the delivery and support of health care services in the United States, both in general terms and by looking at some specific caregiver groups—physicians, nurses, allied health professionals, and the "invisible" caregivers.

Health Manpower Overview

Health care is a "people business," which is defined in a recent *Harvard Business Review* article as a company that has high overall employee costs, exhibits a high ratio of employee costs to capital costs, and engages in a limited number of activities designed to generate future revenue. The focus of the article is on the metrics used to measure productivity, and how the metrics for people businesses must be different from those for businesses whose greatest assets may be raw materials, a finished product, or some other nonhuman commodity. The article identifies the "People Business 40," with IBM and UPS in the lead positions and SAIC (a contract research firm) and WPP (an advertising agency) rounding off the list. At number 5 was HCA, the largest multi-hospital system in the United States, and at number 18 was Tenet Healthcare, another large system. Their inclusion indicates the critical role played by hospital employees in allowing these two giant systems to function—a role that remains significant even when the perspective shifts from a hospital management company to a small rural hospital or to the entire health care delivery system. The article underscores the most basic truth of the health care delivery system: Health care *is* people.[1]

National Overview

In direct contrast to many segments of the U.S. employment market, the health care sector continues to provide a steadily growing source of opportunities for employment and advancement. This trend is almost certain to continue for the foreseeable future, given the increasing needs of a growing senior population combined with the demand by an empowered consumer base for more personalized health care services.

What percentage of the working population is employed in health care?

According to data compiled by the U.S. Bureau of Labor Statistics (BLS), in December 2004 the seasonally adjusted figure for total nonfarm employment in the United States was almost 132.5 million. About 9 percent, or 12.1 million workers, are employed by health care providers. In other words, roughly 1 out of 11 nonfarm workers is employed in the health care field.[2]

What percentage of the working population are employed in hospitals?

Of the 12.1 million people employed in health care, 4.3 million work in hospitals.[3] The hospital

Table 2–1. FTE Personnel in U.S. Registered Hospitals, 1994–2004

Survey Year	Selected Personnel Categories		
	Registered Nurses	Licensed Practical Nurses	Total Personnel
1994	977,765	178,128	4,270,110
1995	980,730	170,130	4,272,815
1996	979,818	165,085	4,276,109
1997	987,404	164,060	4,332,805
1998	1,018,544	160,301	4,406,714
1999	1,022,093	159,043	4,368,638
2000	1,039,994	151,684	4,454,107
2001	1,045,501	153,800	4,535,062
2002	1,073,468	155,863	4,610,206
2003	1,105,251	153,722	4,650,946
2004	1,140,646	150,640	4,695,741

Source: AHA Hospital Statistics, 2006 ed. (Chicago: Health Forum, 2006), and earlier editions.

workforce represents over one-third of all health care employees, and approximately 3.3 percent of the nonfarm workforce.

The American Hospital Association (AHA) also gathers data on the number of hospital employees. The data are reported annually as full-time equivalents (FTEs), a calculation that allows both full- and part-time personnel to be expressed as a single figure. Table 2–1 shows the steady growth that has taken place over a 10-year period in the total number of hospital employees.

Both the BLS and AHA data track only direct employees of hospitals. The tens of thousands of physicians, surgeons, agency-based nurses, and independent contractors who work in hospitals under arrangements other than the traditional employer-employee relationship are not included in these counts.

Local Economy

Hospitals are more than a place where you go to get well. Hospitals are employers, providing good wages and stimulating other areas of business throughout the community. . . . Hospitals truly are the cornerstone of the community.[4]

What role do hospitals play as employers in their communities?

Hospitals are a major presence in the marketplace, whether analyzed aggregately at the national level or examined individually at the local level. This dominance is reflected not only in the number of

hospital employees, but also in the dollar value of the payroll and employee benefits that hospitals contribute to the U.S. economy. In 2003 hospitals spent more than $265 billion dollars on total compensation, a figure representing over 53 percent of their operating expenses.[5] The ripple effect of this expenditure through the local and national economies is substantial.

Several studies have looked at the unique role that rural hospitals play in the communities in which they are located.[6] In a rural community, the local hospital may be one of the largest–if not *the* largest–employer, with consequent impacts on the local economy. The closing of a rural hospital can have a devastating impact not only on the quality and quantity of health care services available to individuals, but also on the overall economic life of the community.

What role do hospitals play in attracting and retaining new businesses and residents to their communities?

Hospitals are economic anchors for the communities they serve. They provide a stable, usually growing, supply of employment opportunities and generally are in a constant state of recruitment and training. Hospital payroll dollars are reinvested in the community through the goods and services purchased by hospital employees. Hospital payrolls contribute to the local tax base through the taxes paid by hospital personnel. Hospitals themselves are also major purchasers of goods and services, contributing to the economic health of local and national vendors.

Like good schools, affordable housing, and convenient shopping, a hospital and the organizations and groups that support it are critical in attracting people to a community. People prefer the availability of high-quality health care services near the areas where they live and work. The local hospital, in providing this care through a combination of on-site services and community outreach programs, is a prominent corporate citizen, integral to the ongoing life of the community it serves.

How can the complex mix of employees and free agents be described?

"The hospital . . . has grown from a marginal institution to which the poor went to die into the center of health care and a giant in its own right–and also into one of the most complex social institutions around."[7] Peter Drucker's often-quoted observation on the intricacies of the modern hospital's infrastructure was made over 30 years ago and has only grown more accurate with the passage of time.

The U.S. Bureau of Labor Statistics lists over 350 job categories for hospital personnel.[8] While it is true that not every hospital employs laboratory animal caretakers, industrial truck operators, or aircraft mechanics, the breadth of employment possibilities available in even the smallest hospitals creates a rich mix of skilled and unskilled workers. Clinical staff with advanced medical or other health-related degrees work side by side with support staff who may have college or high school diplomas. Administrative staff, many with little or no clinical expertise, provide for and maintain the infrastructure that supports the most advanced health care services in the world. A veritable army of support staff moves constantly through the fore- and background of the typical hospital, keeping the floors clean, the linens washed, the food trays delivered, the lights on, and the doors open. This intricate arrangement of interlocking staffs, functions, and responsibilities can best be described as a team, with each person or group possessing a skill or providing a service while simultaneously relying on the skills and services of the other members to move the entire team forward.

How do the clinical and administrative divisions of the hospital work together?

The 1990 National Forum on Hospital and Health Affairs, sponsored by Duke University, was titled *Revisiting the Three-Legged Stool: Striking a New Balance Among Trustees, Administrators, and Physicians.*[9] In the preface to the collection of papers from the forum, B. Jon Jaeger described the "three-legged stool" analogy, postulating that, in an ideal world, the legs would be of equal length (length = power), thus ensuring that the seat would be flat, stable, and functional. Another interpretation of the analogy is a stool where nurses, physicians, and administrators compose the three legs, with hospital trustees balanced on the seat in their governance capacity. In still another variant, the stool becomes a ladder, with physicians and administrators forming the two sides and the board of trustees acting as rungs. Regardless of the model used, the clinical and administrative functions are seen as distinct aspects of the hospital's makeup, with the board acting as either a balance (the third leg of the stool) or a unifying force (the rungs of the ladder).

The ideal of a firmly planted, nicely balanced, three-legged stool falls somewhat short of the reality in many of today's hospitals. In the Institute of Medicine's 2001 landmark report *Crossing the Quality Chasm*, the preeminence given to professional autonomy and the stratification of health care providers into rigid hierarchies are seen as detrimental to the quality of patient care and the efficient functioning of the health care delivery system.[10] The shift from these professional fiefdoms—medical, management, and governance— to a more coordinated team effort is predicated on establishing and maintaining open lines of communications between clinicians, hospital administrators, and the hospital governing board.[11] By engaging in frequent exchanges of information, all three camps acquire a better understanding of the pressures under which each operates and can begin to align their objectives and priorities to the mutual benefit of the patients, the hospital, and themselves.

Health Manpower Issues

Is the workforce shortage brewing up a "perfect storm"?

The supply of health care personnel has always been of great concern, in terms of being either too plentiful or not plentiful enough. Since the end of World War II, the United States has experienced cyclical shortages of health care professionals. These shortages have been the product of a combination of factors, including the economy, alternating pressures on women to be stay-at-home mothers or members of the workforce, and the fluctuating attractiveness of health care occupations, which may rate more highly in a manufacturing economy, but are perceived as less attractive in the current information economy.[12] The last shortage of note prior to the present occurred in the late 1980s, when a deficit of registered nurses became apparent to those monitoring the availability of such personnel.[13] Some believe that this personnel shortage never really ended, and that the crisis now facing hospitals and other health care providers is not part of the normal economic cycle, but has been growing under conditions constituting a "perfect storm" scenario.

Made familiar by a best-selling book and a blockbuster movie, the original "perfect storm" was a real-life meteorological event that occurred in late October 1991. Two storm systems and the lingering remnants of a hurricane came together over the north Atlantic Ocean to create the most powerful storm in recorded history, resulting in 100-foot-high waves and the loss of ships and lives. The analogy of three or more crises combining to create a mega-crisis passed quickly into common parlance and has been used to describe the health care workforce shortage.[14] The scenario can be described as follows:

- A rapidly growing senior population has created increased demand on the health care delivery system for more frequent and complex services.
- The health care delivery system is increasingly financially strapped and must deal with persistent problems of accessibility and quality.
- More personnel are exiting the beleaguered health care delivery system, due to retirement and career change, than are entering as new graduates or recruits from other work sectors.

From such ingredients are perfect storms created.

The advances made in medical, biomedical, and other health-related sciences during the last 50 years border on the fabulous when compared with the practice of medicine at the beginning of the twentieth century. Many of the new technologies demand highly trained personnel with specific skills in operating diagnostic equipment, interpreting laboratory tests down to the level of the code embedded in human DNA, or delivering innovative therapies both in the traditional inpatient setting and in the more flexible environment of outpatient services. The requirements of high-tech medicine have resulted in personnel shortages in allied health occupations, including pharmacists, radiology/nuclear imaging technologists, respiratory therapists, and laboratory technicians, as well as physical and occupational therapists, all registering double-digit vacancy rates in the latest *Health Care Metrics Study*[15] from the Bernard Hodes Group.

There is grave concern that the lack of appropriately trained and adequately distributed health care personnel is having a direct impact on the quality of health care and patient safety. Numerous studies are examining the effects of heavy workloads on the incidence of medical errors, conditions that could not be treated in a timely manner, and hospital-acquired illnesses and infections.[16] There is also research addressing the more subtle, but no less damaging, impact of inadequate staffing on job performance, morale, and staff loyalty.[17]

In light of these studies, hospitals and other health care providers are actively engaged in creating work environments that emphasize safety, ensure quality, and encourage both new employees and seasoned workers to remain in health care. Since 2002 the AHA Commission on Workforce has issued a series of reports that provide some background on the causes and impacts of the current crisis, but focus primarily on case studies of recruitment programs, employee involvement and recognition programs, community and academic partnerships, and other initiatives implemented by hospitals around the country to maintain their current complement of employees and to nurture the next generation of health care service providers.[18]

Why is diversity a critical issue?

As a nation, the U.S. population represents the most comprehensive amalgamation of ethnic and racial groups in the history of mankind. Hospitals are called upon to provide care to this population at a very intimate level, consequently encountering a bewildering array of cultural mores, taboos, practices, languages, religious beliefs, and prejudices that must be acknowledged and addressed to ensure optimal health outcomes. A workforce that is itself culturally, ethnically, and racially diverse is best positioned to respond with sensitivity and understanding to the individual needs of patients, effectively utilizing cultural and ethnic tools to promote healing and health.

While there has been measurable progress on this front in the recent past, the ethnic and racial mix of the current health care workforce does not yet reflect that of the general population. For example, data from the most recent National Sample Survey of Registered Nurses, conducted every four years by the U.S. Bureau of Health Professions, indicate that the numbers of African American and Hispanic nurses rose more dramatically between 1986 and 2000 than in any other four-year period since 1980. However, in 2000 the majority of nurses, 69 percent, were white. Although people of Hispanic ancestry constitute 12.5 percent of the general population, Hispanics account for only 2 percent of all registered nurses.[19] To ensure an adequate supply of caregivers and support staff, it is imperative that hospitals and other health care providers broaden their hiring efforts by reaching out to ethnic and racial groups currently underrepresented in the health care workforce. This initiative also entails breaking away from the traditional perspective of the predominantly female-oriented role of caregiver and attracting more men into the nursing and allied health professions.

How serious is the malpractice crisis?

Since 1990 the *Medical Liability Monitor* has conducted an annual survey of premiums paid by physicians for malpractice insurance, tracking the rise and fall (but mostly rise) of these rates by specialty and state. The latest data, published in the October 2004 issue, offer a glimmer of hope: The usually skyrocketing rise of annual premium rates had diminished somewhat compared with previous years' increases. There were more instances of either no change or even negative change (i.e., a rate that had dropped) from the previous year. At the same time, there were more instances of rates increasing 100 percent or more—the most dramatic case being reported for Maryland's obstetricians and gynecologists, who in 2004 were paying almost 133 percent more in premiums than they had paid in 2003. While the premium juggernaut may be slowing, rates are still prohibitively high and are likely to remain so for the foreseeable future.[20]

Fueling the rise in malpractice premiums are the awards being granted in malpractice cases. In 2003 the average court-ordered payment was $4,723,425. The good news is that this dollar amount represented a reduction of almost 15 percent from the previous year. The bad news is that the range of awards, from smallest to largest, was $5,000 to $112 million, the uppermost value representing an increase of over 18 percent from 2002.[21] While it is true that most malpractice claims are settled out of court, the possibility of having to pay out on one or more multi–million-dollar lawsuits has created enough pressure for liability insurance companies to raise their rates in direct correlation to the prospects of huge losses. Some companies have stopped offering insurance policies in specific states, while others have either restricted their underwriting policies or simply gotten out of the first-line insurance business altogether.[22]

The reality of unaffordable or unavailable malpractice insurance and the risk of catastrophic financial losses from even one malpractice suit have forced many physicians to give up their medical practices or to move to states where tort reform has had a mitigating impact on such losses. In states with no mandate on a minimum level of insurance, some physicians choose to "go bare," that is, either forgo commercial insurance or become self-insured. Some hospitals have eased or eliminated long-standing policies requiring medical staff to carry liability coverage. In many cases, "going bare" is the only way for a specialist to continue practicing medicine in a hostile malpractice insurance environment.

The impact of the liability crisis on hospitals is no less staggering than the impact on individual physicians. Hospitals must also contend with costly insurance premiums, both those paid to cover the hospital's own liability and those paid for physicians whom the hospital has decided to cover under its own or a separate policy. Beyond the dollars devoted to managing liability coverage, however, hospitals face a more serious problem. With physicians leaving to practice medicine elsewhere, or leaving the practice of medicine altogether, hospitals in certain "crisis" states are experiencing grave difficulties in recruiting physicians and offering certain high-risk services such as obstetrics and emergency medicine.[23]

Health Care Professions

Caring for the sick, injured, and dying is not a light-hearted job description, and yet every day, millions of hospital and health care workers do just that. This section will examine the most visible of the health care professionals—physicians, nurses, and the allied health professions—as well as the "invisible" caregivers: those individuals who provide care outside the formal structure of the health care delivery system.

Physicians

In 2003 the American Medical Association reported that there were 871,535 physicians in the United States.[24] An overwhelming majority (79 percent) of these physicians were engaged in direct patient care—most in office-based practice, but some in hospital-based practice, either as residents or as full-time staff physicians. Other professional activities included administration, teaching, and research. The American Osteopathic Association reported an additional 54,000-plus osteopathic physicians.[25]

What is the difference between allopathic and osteopathic physicians?

Most physicians in the United States can be classified as allopathic. *Mosby's Medical, Nursing, & Allied Health Dictionary* defines an allopathic physician as one who treats illnesses and injuries through active interventions that are designed to counteract the effects of those illnesses and injuries. Active interventions include medical and surgical treatments.[26]

Osteopathic medicine, as it is currently practiced, uses many of the same diagnostic and treatment techniques employed by allopathic physicians. There is, however, a greater emphasis on the relationship of the body's structure—nerves, muscle tissue, and bones—to illness and injury. Osteopathic manipulative treatment, often referred to simply as OMT, is used both diagnostically and therapeutically, and also has applications in preventive medicine. OMT involves the osteopathic physician's use of the hands to administer stretching, gentle pressure, or resistance to muscles and joints.[27]

All physicians, regardless of whether they practice allopathic or osteopathic medicine, must complete four years of medical school and additional years of residency training in their chosen specialty, must be licensed to practice by the state, and must complete continuing medical education courses throughout their careers.

Is there a physician shortage?

Expert opinion suggests that the United States is either on the verge of or in the early stages of a physician shortage. The Council on Graduate Medical Education (COGME) released a report in January 2005 predicting a shortfall of 85,000 doctors by 2020 unless its recommendations are followed.[28] The report effectively reversed the position that COGME, an advisory group authorized by Congress to monitor and report on trends in the physician workforce, had held for more than a decade. Other studies have employed a variety of methodologies to measure current and future physician demand and workload, and the predicted shortfalls expand or contract accordingly, but most observers agree that a shortage exists and will worsen unless changes are made in medical education and physician distribution.

While there are many ways to measure supply and demand, one of the most commonly used metrics is the physician/population ratio. A frequently cited study of physician/population ratios was conducted by the Graduate Medical Education National Advisory Committee (GMENAC).[29] The final recommendations of the GMENAC study were issued in 1981 and are still used today for everything from forecasting physician demand at the national level to creating a medical staff five-year development plan for an individual hospital. A succinct overview of various physician/population ratio studies, from GMENAC to the present, is provided by H.J. Simmons and John M. Harris in the December 2004 issue of *Health Care Strategic Management*.[30]

The distribution of physicians is uneven across the country. The U.S. Bureau of Health Professions uses the tagline "The right people, with the right skills, in the right places, to achieve the right health outcomes." To achieve this level of "rightness," the bureau identifies geographic areas and/or populations that fall into one of three categories: health professional shortage area (HPSA), medically underserved area (MUA), or medically underserved population (MUP). There are almost three dozen federal assistance programs that use these shortage designations to determine eligibility or funding priority.

Health professional shortage areas have shortages of primary medical care, dental, and/or mental health providers and may be urban or rural areas, population groups, or certain medical or other public facilities. About 20 percent of the U.S. population live in an area designated as an HPSA. A medically underserved area may be an entire county or a group of contiguous counties, a group of county or civil divisions, or a group of urban census tracts in which the residents face a shortage of personal health services. A medically underserved population may include groups of individuals who confront economic, cultural, or linguistic barriers to health care. More extensive information about shortage areas—where they are located and how they are designated—can be found at the bureau's website.[31]

Are there too many specialists?

Complicating the issue of adequate and equitable distribution of physicians is that of clinical specialization. Items of concern here are how much specialization the health care delivery system requires to ensure high-quality care, how many physicians are needed in each specialty, and how these specialists should be distributed among the general population for optimal service delivery.

Physicians can be categorized as primary care physicians (PCPs)—general and family practice, general internal medicine, general pediatrics—or as specialists. The evolution of high-tech medicine has brought a corresponding proliferation of highly focused areas of practice, some boasting only a handful of practitioners. The American Board of Medical Specialties includes 24 approved medical specialty certification boards under its corporate umbrella. Of these 24 boards, 18 offer subspecialty certificates in a total of 86 practice areas.[32] The AMA counted 185 self-designated specialties in its latest analysis of the physician population.[33] That same analysis showed that out of 871,535 physicians, there were 525,096 (60 percent) whose main practice was in a specialty.[34]

Specialists are unevenly distributed in the United States; they are concentrated in urban and suburban settings, leaving large segments of the rural population without easy access to certain specialty services.[35] The hazards inherent in a health care system that emphasizes specialization over adequate supplies of primary care physicians are spelled out in studies that reveal a positive correlation between the number of PCPs and the well-being of the general population.[36] On the other hand, people who visit a physician's office are just as likely to visit a specialist as they are to visit a primary care physician. In 2002, 54 percent of all physician office visits were to primary care physicians and 46 percent were to specialists. Visits to obstetricians/gynecologists accounted for 8 percent of the visits to specialists.[37]

There is no simple answer to the question of whether there are too many specialists. Any attempts to develop a more appropriate distribution of specialists based on population or health service needs will require an extensive reorganization and reprioritization of graduate medical education, physician incentives, and health care policy and planning in general. It will also necessitate fundamental shifts in the mindset of physicians on the verge of choosing a specialty and in the preferences of the general population who have grown accustomed to being treated by specialists as a matter of course.

What are the implications of increasing numbers of women physicians?

In 1849 Elizabeth Blackwell graduated from the Geneva Medical College in New York, becoming the first woman to earn a medical degree from an American medical school. She and her sister Emily, who graduated from Western Reserve University's medical school in 1854, founded the New York Infirmary for Women and Children in New York City and, in 1867, established a medical college for women.[38] Since those pioneering times, women have gradually swelled the ranks of physicians in the United States. According to the American Medical Association, there were about 225,000 female physicians in 2003, representing about one-fourth of all physicians. By 2010 women may represent as much as one-third of the physician population.[39]

The nearly continuous growth in the female physician population has had an inevitable, if somewhat uneven, impact on the practice of medicine. Studies have attempted to identify and analyze the male/female differential of medical practice, including the preference of female physicians for certain specialties, such as obstetrics/gynecology, pediatrics, and internal medicine;[40] the different styles of communication that female physicians employ with their patients;[41] the effect of physician gender on patient satisfaction;[42] and the professional advancement of women in medical academia.[43] The Venus/Mars dichotomy manifests itself in virtually every aspect of practice, and it is doubtful that a true quantification is possible.

Does the physician population reflect the diversity of the nation?

While the role played by women in the medical profession has, for the most part, expanded over time, the same is not true for physicians from ethnic and racial minority groups. Table 2–2 shows the distribution of both the general and physician populations in the United States by race. While a definitive analysis is not possible, given the fact that over a third of the physicians surveyed by the AMA did not identify their racial/ethnic origin, the data that are available tend to support the hypothesis that the current physician population does not reflect the diversity of the general population.

An analysis of students graduating from U.S. medical schools does not provide an optimistic

Table 2–2. Distribution of Physicians by Race Compared with U.S. Resident Population, 2003		
Race	U.S. Resident Population	Physicians
White	67.9	49.0
African American	12.8	2.4
Hispanic	13.7	3.3
Asian	4.1	8.4
American/Alaska Native	0.96	0.1
Other	0.61	2.3
Unknown	n/a	34.0

Statistical Abstract of the United States: 2004–2005. (Washington, DC: Census Bureau, 2005), 15. http://www.census.gov/prod/2004pubs/04statab/pop.pdf (accessed May 6, 2005); *Physician Characteristics and Distribution in the US,* 2005 ed. (Chicago: American Medical Association, 2005), 43.

outlook for a culturally diverse physician population. Data collected by the Association of American Medical Colleges (AAMC) show that graduates from underrepresented minority groups (defined by AAMC as U.S. citizens or permanent residents who identify themselves as African American, American/Alaska Native, Native Hawaiian, Mexican American, or mainland Puerto Rican on their medical school applications) have represented just over 10 percent of medical school graduates since the 1995–1996 school year.[44] The U.S. Census Bureau anticipates that as a percentage of the overall population, ethnic and racial minority groups will continue to increase at least until 2050, with a simultaneous decrease in the white population.[45] Unless medical schools can find a way to recruit and nurture minority students, the "diversity gap" between physicians and the patients they serve will continue to widen.

The importance of a culturally diverse complement of physicians cannot be overstated. A position paper developed by the American College of Physicians (ACP) on racial and ethnic disparities in health care posits as one of its main tenets that "[a] diverse workforce of health professionals is an important part of eliminating disparities among racial and ethnic minorities."[46] The paper cites research identifying a positive correlation between a physician's minority status and the number of minority, uninsured, and Medicaid patients that the physician treats. A subsequent comment on the ACP position paper, while questioning the airtightness of the argument that diversity dispels disparity, does acknowledge the logic of the argument and cites several studies that support the ACP findings.[47]

What is the current status and source of reimbursement for graduate medical education?

Medical students are not the only bearers of the high costs involved in ensuring a well-educated physician workforce. Academic medical centers and other teaching hospitals provide a "classroom of experience" in which doctors become immersed in direct patient care and, in many instances, clinical research. These facilities also provide highly specialized, technology-intensive patient care. From its inception, Medicare recognized the enhanced quality of care provided in an academic environment, as well as the attendant costs, and in 1985 the Consolidated Omnibus Budget Reconciliation Act (often referred to as COBRA) and its subsequent

regulations established a methodology for reimbursing teaching hospitals for the expenses incurred in providing a learning environment for medical residents. Medicare remains the primary source of medical education payments, both direct (for such things as resident and faculty salaries) and indirect (for the more intangible costs of maintaining the academic mission of the hospital), with some additional funds coming from private payors. Both direct and indirect payments are calculated using multipliers based on the number of residents training at the hospital, as well as a measure of the hospital's Medicare volume—either patient days or discharges.

Some of the current tensions surrounding direct and indirect medical education payments relate to the formula used to calculate full-time–equivalent residents (only those involved in direct patient care and only those hours devoted to direct patient care are eligible) and the availability of funds to reimburse children's teaching hospitals, which, almost by definition, do not often treat Medicare-eligible patients. A letter submitted in April 2004 by the AHA to the chairman of the House Appropriations Subcommittee, Labor, Health and Human Services, and Education, highlighted the critical role children's hospitals play in graduate medical education (GME): "Although they represent less than one percent of all hospitals, independent children's teaching hospitals train almost 30 percent of all pediatricians, almost half of all pediatric subspecialists, and two-thirds of pediatric critical care physicians. Equitable GME funding for children's hospitals is a sound investment in the future of children's health."[48]

What happened to physician practice management companies?

Physician practice management companies (PPMC) came into vogue in the 1990s as a way to organize physician practices into larger units to achieve economies of scale, obtain access to capital, and negotiate for managed-care contracts.[49] Many of the PPMCs were newly formed for-profit companies that banked on their ability to efficiently manage physician practices and create shareholder value in the process. The collapse of the PPMC market was due in large part to the aggressive practice acquisition programs executed by companies such as PhyCor, MedPartners, and PhyMatrix and their subsequent failure to integrate the acquired practices into a smoothly operating enterprise. The much-heralded administrative efficiencies never materialized, the projected improved operating margins and profits never resulted, stock prices and earnings per share tanked, and the market boom for PPMCs ended with several companies filing for bankruptcy or being delisted from the stock exchanges.[50]

Not all PPMCs vanished when the bubble burst. Pediatrix is a good example of a PPMC that survived the market shakeout by carving a well-defined niche—hospital-based neonatology—and demonstrating a true ability to create value-added services for the physicians in its acquired practices. EmCare, a PPMC focused on emergency medicine, currently has 4,500 physicians providing care in over 300 hospital emergency departments. Per-Se Technologies offers a service called MedAxxis, a physician practice management package that draws on the company's expertise in front-office efficiencies and revenue cycle management. In 1997, at the height of the PPMC glory days, approximately 16 percent of medical group practices were managed by or affiliated with a PPMC; by 2001 the figure had dwindled to around 2.5 percent.[51] The companies remaining in the market now operate in a less glamorous, but also less volatile, environment.

How is physician practice changing?

After several decades characterized by various attempts to level the playing field of health care through managed-care and government programs, the pendulum has begun to swing the other way. "Concierge" medicine, "boutique" practice, and "retainer-based" practice are the terms applied to the latest development in medical practice, in which a physician or group practice deliberately limits service to a fixed number of patients (600 to 800 seems to be the most common range), a practice calculated to allow them to deliver highly personalized and timely care while generating an adequate revenue stream. The patients seen by physicians in these arrangements pay a fixed sum up front, ranging from $1,000 per individual to $20,000 for a couple, exclusive of actual medical costs; in return they can expect appointments, scheduled on a same-day or next-day basis, that may last 30 minutes or longer; physicians who may make house calls; and other personalized services.[52] The retainer fee does not take the place of traditional health insurance; rather, the fee ensures a more personalized level of physician care for the person willing and able to pay it.

Discussions about concierge medicine tend to involve issues of ethics and morality. While these practices can be seen as a natural outgrowth of the American entrepreneurial spirit, they are also condemned as elitist and contributing to the widening gap between the haves and have-nots in a health care system that already bears a heavy burden of uninsured and underinsured. The impact of concierge medicine on the health care delivery system may be more hypothetical than real since the number of physicians actually engaged in these practices is very small; however, the very existence of concierge medicine does force consideration of what we envision as the future model of health care delivery in the United States.

How do hospitals and physicians work together?

Although the medical profession predates the development of hospitals by millennia, it is hard to imagine one without the other in today's health care model. As the two dominant forces in the delivery of health care, physicians and hospitals are highly interdependent, while at the same time competing with each other for patients and revenue. Relations between hospitals and physicians move back and forth on the cooperation-competition continuum. Today's environment appears to fall more in the range of cooperation in the interest of mutual survival.

Joint ventures allow the two diametrically opposed aspects of cooperation and competition in the hospital-physician relation to come together to the advantage of both parties. Joint ventures are as varied as the hospitals and physicians that create them. Some of the common models are medical office buildings, ambulatory surgery centers or other types of freestanding outpatient facilities, group purchasing organizations, integrated centers of excellence, and exclusive contracts between hospitals and specialty practices, such as cardiology or radiology. Looming over all such arrangements are antitrust considerations, as well as the Stark laws—named after U.S. Representative Fortney "Pete" Stark, D-California, an influential crusader in the struggle to eliminate health care fraud and abuse, and chairman of the House Ways and Means Subcommittee on Health during the late 1980s—which were designed to inhibit a physician's ability to refer Medicare and Medicaid patients for certain designated health services to other health care providers in which the physician or a member of the physician's family has a financial interest. Chapter 5 includes additional information on the Stark laws (see the section "Ethics in Patient Referrals Act").

Even without the benefit of a formal joint-venture arrangement, a hospital's medical staff wields enormous economic influence. First and foremost, the medical staff admit and treat patients, which allows the hospital to fulfill its healing mission. The composition of the medical staff and the availability of specialists dictate the type and level of services provided by the hospital, including its qualification as a trauma center and the designated level of its neonatal intensive care unit.[53] The medical staff help create and maintain the hospital's presence and reputation within the community, while the hospital markets the medical staff to the community by offering physician referral and other services.

Gain sharing is being explored as a means of leveraging economics to create stronger ties between the hospital and medical staff. One gain sharing model that shows promise has evolved in materials management; specialists, such as cardiologists or orthopedic surgeons, agree to draw from a mutually agreed-upon list of medical devices and equipment, thereby limiting the number of vendors with which the hospital's purchasing department must contend, and increasing the volume of orders placed with those vendors with which the hospital continues to do business. Savings from a more efficient purchasing program are not only realized but shared between the hospital and the involved physicians. As with joint ventures, there are sensitive legal issues involved in the development of gain sharing programs, but both the DHHS Office of Inspector General and the Medicare Payment Advisory Commission have recently shown signs of supporting such arrangements.[54]

A more intimate level of interdependence between hospitals and physicians is forged when the medical staff become integrated into the hospital's governance structure. The Governance Institute's latest biennial survey of hospital and health system governance structure found that just under 90 percent of respondents have physicians on the governing board.[55] A shared vision of the hospital and its mission can be nurtured by medical staff leadership through the creation of opportunities for such functions as sitting on the hospital board, serving on the strategic planning committee, participating in a capital fund-raising campaign, or taking on the administrative responsibilities of vice president of medical affairs, chief of medical staff, or head of a clinical service line.

Physician involvement with hospital management has sometimes extended beyond the role of medical staff to owner status. It is not unheard of for a group of physicians to pool their resources toward the purchase of a hospital that is on the verge of closing or to open a new hospital where one did not previously exist. Physician ownership of hospitals and other types of health facilities falls squarely on the thin line separating cooperation and competition, and a relatively recent development in the marketplace—special (or specialty) hospitals—further attests to the delicate balance between the two.

How do hospitals and physicians compete against each other?

Competition between community hospitals and physicians arises from physician ownership of limited-service hospitals and ambulatory care facilities. Limited-service hospitals, which will be discussed in greater detail in chapter 3, have proliferated since the early 1990s. Specialty hospitals, such as children's hospitals or rehabilitation institutes, have been in operation for many years. Physicians have had ownership interests in hospitals in the past; what differentiates the new generation of limited-service hospitals is their focus on service lines, such as cardiology or orthopedic surgery, that are often key centers of excellence in, and important sources of revenue for, the local full-service community hospital. Loss of market share in these signature service lines makes it more difficult for community hospitals to provide essential services, such as emergency departments or burn units, which are seldom self-supporting.[56]

A not-so-new source of competitive tension between hospitals and physicians, specifically surgeons, is the booming outpatient surgery market. For many years, it was the accepted wisdom that surgery of any kind was best and most safely performed in a hospital setting. With the advent of less invasive techniques, more effective postoperative pharmaceuticals, the pressure exerted by inadequate reimbursement for hospital stays, and the growing demand from both consumers and physicians for greater convenience, much of the surgical volume has shifted to hospital-based or freestanding ambulatory surgery centers and physician offices. The latest data from the National Center for Health Statistics (NCHS) indicates that in 2002, physicians ordered or performed nearly 69.8 million surgical procedures. NCHS estimates that approximately 45 percent of these procedures were performed in physicians' offices.[57] As outpatient surgical volume increases, so does the number of venues in which such procedures are performed, and hospitals must compete with local physicians and surgeons, as well as national chains of ambulatory surgery centers, to maintain adequate levels of service and revenue.

Are hospitalists a fad?

The Society of Hospital Medicine, the professional society of hospitalists, defines the specialty as "physicians whose primary professional focus is the general medical care of hospitalized patients. Their activities include patient care, teaching, research, and leadership related to Hospital Medicine."[58] Although the term *hospitalist* did not come into widespread use until the mid-1990s, the actual practice of using designated physicians exclusively to handle inpatients was first implemented almost a decade earlier by large multi-specialty practices.[59]

The number of practitioners of this new specialty has grown exponentially. In 2000 the society estimated that there were around 1,000 hospitalists; five years later the estimate now hovers around 12,000, and as many as 30,000 hospitalists may be practicing by 2010.[60] Hospitalists have quickly passed from fad to the emerging model of inpatient care for the new millennium, and it is estimated that approximately half of all U.S. academic and community hospitals with 200 or more beds have a hospitalist program in place.[61]

What is the role of physician extenders?

Physician extenders, or nonphysician clinicians, are health care professionals who are licensed and/or certified to provide defined levels of health care services. Professionals who have developed the capacity to act as physician extenders include physician assistants and advanced practice nurses, including nurse midwives and nurse anesthetists. Physician extenders increase the capacity of the health care system to manage service demand volume by virtue of their ability to meet with, diagnose, treat, and, for some professions, prescribe drugs for patients who might otherwise go without care due to an inadequate supply of physicians. In a typical practice setting, physician assistants and advanced practice nurses may also increase staff physicians' ability to concentrate on those patients with more complex medical needs by handling the bulk of demand for primary care services, thus creating a more efficient and productive delivery model.

Tensions linger, however, between physicians and these "extender" professions. Providing prescribing privileges for physician assistants and nurse practitioners, while authorized by law, was a hotly contested, state-by-state struggle, and nurse anesthetists still battle with anesthesiologists over reimbursement for unsupervised anesthesia practice.[62] Only time will tell if the growth in the number of physician extenders and the expansion of their respective scopes of professional practice has improved the overall efficiency and quality of the health care system, or has simply led to more fragmentation of service delivery and professional conflicts with physicians.

Nurses

Patients want empathy, anticipation of their needs and a personalized, humanized experience—something that nurses do every day. Nurses clearly influence patient satisfaction, but more subtly, their ability to work with other people on the care team influences the patient's perception of the hospital. How nurses project their joys or frustrations can influence how patients feel about the things they don't see in the hospital.[63]

How many nurses are there in the United States?

There are several major occupational categories that use the word *nurse*, such as licensed practical nurse, licensed vocational nurse, nurse aid, and nurse assistant. The focus of this section is on registered nurses, that is, those individuals who have successfully completed a course of study at a state-approved school of nursing and passed the National Council Licensure Examination.[64] Registered nurses constitute the largest health care profession in the United States; data from the U.S. Bureau of Labor Statistics showed a total of 2.3 million RNs as of May 2004.[65] The American Nurses Association describes itself as representing 2.7 million nurses, no doubt including individuals not counted in the BLS data: the self-employed, retired, unemployed, and nurses employed in non-nursing positions.[66]

How many nurses practice in hospitals?

The 2004 AHA Annual Survey indicated that there were 1.1 million full-time–equivalent RNs working in U.S. hospitals, as shown in table 2–1. The U.S. Bureau of Labor Statistics data indicate that hospitals are the largest employers of RNs by a huge margin, accounting for over 57 percent of the RNs included in the survey; the next largest employer of RNs are physicians' offices, representing almost 9 percent of the RN working population. Nursing homes and home health agencies each account for about 5 percent.[67]

How much are nurses paid?

The nursing staff in a hospital is a complex mix of positions, levels of expertise, areas of specialization, and years of experience. Salary structures are usually based on formulas that factor in all these variables, allowing for great variation in compensation packages among U.S. hospitals. Salary offerings are also affected by whether the hospital is independent or part of a multi-hospital system, under what type of ownership the facility operates (government, for-profit, not-for-profit), whether it is a teaching hospital, where the hospital is located (urban, suburban, rural), and how many beds it has.

The *Hospital Compensation Report*, an annual report produced by the Hay Group, is based on the results of a salary and benefits survey conducted on behalf of the American Society for Healthcare Human Resources Administration. In addition to two executive nursing positions (top patient care executive/top nursing executive and head of nursing services/director of nursing), the survey includes 15 nursing positions, plus data for licensed practical nurses. Table 2–3 provides compensation data for a selected number of these positions.

What does it take to be competitive in attracting nurses?

It is no secret that hospitals compete against each other—for patients, for physicians, and for staff, most visibly nurses. The current workforce shortage "perfect storm"—an increasing demand for health services, an overextended delivery system, and a decreasing supply of health care providers—has forced hospitals and their recruiting personnel to develop a more holistic understanding of the issues involved in staffing to capacity. No longer are hospitals focused solely on recruitment strategies, such as signing bonuses or relocation packages, to fill vacant positions. Hospital recruiters, as well as hospital executives in human resources, nursing, strategic planning, and other key areas, are now looking for those strategies, partnerships, and programs that will ensure an adequate supply of educated and skilled health care workers to fill positions that will be vacant 5 and 10 years from now. In some places, like Columbus, Ohio, hospitals and hospital systems are pooling their recruitment efforts—exchanging competition for collaboration—in order to attract health care workers to their area over a long period of time.[68]

One of the major focuses of this new holistic approach to recruitment has been identifying effective strategies to encourage young people to give serious thought to the health care professions. The AHA Commission on Workforce's 2002 report *In Our Hands* underscored the importance of this

Table 2–3. Annual Base Salary for Selected Nursing Positions

Position	Lowest	Median	Average	Highest
Top patient care/nursing executive	$100,700	$138,800	$141,100	$185,100
Head of nursing services/DON	$81,800	$99,600	$101,400	$124,700
Nurse manager/head nurse	$62,600	$77,600	$77,800	$93,800
Nurse supervisor	$54,700	$67,700	$68,900	$85,500
Charge nurse	$51,700	$62,900	$63,900	$79,400
RN: Level 1	$42,800	$49,900	$51,000	$61,500
RN: Level 2	$45,800	$54,100	$55,400	$66,200
RN: Level 3	$50,100	$61,200	$60,500	$69,800
RN: Level 4	$55,900	$66,800	$68,700	$100,000
RN: Operating room, level 1	$45,100	$55,300	$55,200	$64,700
RN: Operating room, level 2	$52,200	$58,800	$59,400	$69,200
RN: Operating room, level 3	$58,700	$63,400	$64,600	$75,500
Infection control nurse	$50,500	$59,900	$61,400	$75,100
Nurse practitioner	$64,100	$74,400	$75,900	$88,800
Clinical nurse specialist	$55,700	$68,500	$69,400	$85,300
Nurse anesthetist	$115,400	$129,300	$130,200	$146,400

Source: Hay Group, "Section A: Hospital Management Positions"; "Section B: Nursing Positions," *Hospital Compensation Report*, 2005 ed. (Philadelphia: Hay Group, 2005), copyright © 2005 Hay Acquisition Company I, Inc. All rights reserved.

effort, making it one of five major recommendations. Health career academies and mentoring programs offered to local high school students, partnerships with local college and university nursing programs to develop competency guidelines for new graduates or to supply faculty from the hospital staff, partnerships with corporations and foundations to launch campaigns to attract young people to health care—these are just some of the activities in which hospitals are engaging to ensure their future viability.[69]

One of the more recent developments in attracting and retaining nursing staff is the "magnet hospital" designation. Magnet status is conferred by the Commission on Magnet Recognition of the American Nurses Credentialing Center. The term comes from a 1983 study by the American Academy of Nursing task force on hospital nursing practice that identified variables contributing to a hospital's ability to attract and retain nurses.[70] These variables were referred to as "forces of magnetism," and hospitals exhibiting these forces were called magnet hospitals. The forces of magnetism include quality of nursing leadership, organizational structure, management style, personnel policies and programs, professional models of care, quality of care, quality improvement, consultation and resources, autonomy, community-hospital relations, nurses as teachers, image of nursing, interdisciplinary relationships, and professional development.[71] The first magnet hospitals were designated in 1990. As of June 2005 there were 141 magnet hospitals in the United States and one in Australia.[72] Magnet hospitals undergo a rigorous evaluation by a team of specially trained appraisers and must reapply for magnet status every four years.

How are RNs trained today?

Basic nursing education is offered in three settings: the diploma program, the associate degree, and the baccalaureate degree. The diploma program is a two- to three-year course of study offered by hospital-based schools of nursing. The number of these programs has declined dramatically: The 1995 edition of the *AHA Guide* listed 117 hospital schools of nursing, but the 2005 edition included only 9.[73] Associate degrees are also two- to three-year programs, usually in a junior college or community college setting, with additional non-nursing requirements such as basic science and English coursework. The baccalaureate program is the traditional four-year college program with a major in nursing and conferring either a BSN or a BS.

Graduates from all three nursing programs are eligible for the National Council Licensure Examination. One of the many ironies of the workforce shortage crisis is that over 32,000 qualified applicants for baccalaureate and graduate nursing programs for the 2004–2005 academic year were denied admission due to faculty shortages and/or constrained resources.[74]

According to the U.S. Bureau of Health Professions 2000 survey, approximately 40 percent of RNs held an associate degree in nursing, with the other 60 percent divided almost equally between diploma programs and baccalaureate programs. When the analysis was limited to nurses who graduated in the period 1996–2000, the percentage of RNs with associate degrees rose to 55 percent, baccalaureate degrees accounted for 38 percent, and diploma programs were responsible for only 6 percent.[75]

Beyond the basic nursing education that all RNs must complete, around 10 percent go on to complete master's or doctoral degrees in nursing or nursing-related fields.[76] There are also programs that offer advanced training in a particular clinical field without conferring a degree; many advanced practice nurses complete this type of educational program. Nurses whose initial education was completed in a hospital-based nursing school or a junior college may now participate in fast-track baccalaureate programs designed specifically to assist them in acquiring the credits they need to be awarded a bachelor's degree. Finally, like physicians and many other health care professionals, nurses are required to complete continuing education courses on an ongoing basis in order to maintain their licenses and/or certifications.

Is the RN workforce aging?

The RN workforce has been aging steadily in recent years, both in terms of the average age of RNs generally and in the average age of new graduates from basic nursing education programs. In 1980 a new graduate with an associate's degree was, on average, 28 years old; in 2000 the average age of that new graduate was 33. In 1980, 25 percent of RNs were under the age of 30; in 2000, RNs under the age of 30 accounted for only 9 percent.[77]

The RN employment picture becomes even more alarming when data at the other end of the age spectrum are considered. Nurses are leaving the profession, either through retirement, death, or career change, at a higher rate than ever before. The decline in the number of RNs between 1988 and 1992 was 30,000, and the number actually declined to 23,000 between the 1992 and 1996 surveys. However, the number of RNs leaving nursing shot up to 175,000 between 1996 and 2000. There are approximately 500,000 licensed RNs who are not employed as nurses in any capacity.[78] The very real fear of nursing societies and health care providers alike is that as nurses retire, die, or find employment (or unemployment) outside of health care, the drain on the pool of employable RNs will continue to exceed the rate of replenishment.

One aspect of the age factor affecting the nurse population that is more pronounced today than ever before is the distinct profile of characteristics distinguishing members of one generation from those of another. The cover article in the March 2005 issue of *Hospitals & Health Networks* segmented the RN workforce into four generational "camps": matures/veterans/silent generation (born 1922 to 1943); Baby Boomers (born 1943 to 1960); Generation X (born 1960 to 1980); and Generation Y/"Nexters" (born 1980 or later). Each camp displays its own set of characteristics, often placing them at odds with the other groups. For example, nurse veterans, many about to end their careers, tend to place a higher value on paying one's dues and on a long-term commitment to one employer than their youngest colleagues, who are more likely to shop around for the employment situation that best matches their work/life expectations.[79] For their part, hospitals must find ways to make themselves attractive to these young RNs while also identifying effective strategies to retain older, more seasoned RNs, and must encourage the camps to work together as a seamless patient care team.

Why is mandatory overtime such a hot-button issue?

Nursing shortages, staff scheduling needs, 24/7 patient care coverage, quality of care, patient safety, worker safety—these are just some of the ingredients in the volatile mix underlying the issue of mandatory overtime. Mandatory overtime, the enforced scheduling of overtime hours to cover gaps in staffing, is opposed by the American Nurses Association. The ANA prefaced its 2001 opposition statement by summarizing the effects of such overtime in the face of inadequate staffing: "Inadequate staffing is a source of nurses' job dissatisfaction, further contributing to the problem of recruitment and retention of nurses, and with

the attraction of new talent to the profession. The absence of prohibitions or limitations on overtime work may contribute to health care errors, as well as work-related illnesses and injuries among nursing staff."[80] A study headed by researchers at the University of Pennsylvania School of Nursing revealed a significant increase in the number of errors committed by hospital staff nurses working shifts longer than 12 hours.[81]

The U.S. Department of Labor's Fair Labor Standards Act requires employers to pay nonexempt employees for any overtime, defined as all time worked beyond 40 hours in any given work week. Despite the fact that many nurses are paid on an hourly, as opposed to a salary, basis, they have long been considered exempt because of their status as "learned professional employees."[82] In 2004 the weekly salary ceiling for determining nonexempt status was raised for the first time in 50 years, from $155 to $455. There was some concern on the part of nursing groups that hospitals would reclassify their nurses as exempt and force them to work overtime without the benefit of overtime pay. As of April 2005, this prospect had not materialized.[83]

Legislation limiting or banning mandatory overtime has been proposed in half the states; to date, California, Connecticut, Maine, Maryland, Minnesota, New Jersey, Oregon, Texas, Washington, and West Virginia have enacted such proposals.[84] While none of the proposed or enacted legislation has been aimed at limiting voluntary overtime, the research results are clear on the hazards of working shifts longer than half a day; and even in its opposition to mandatory overtime, the American Nurses Association does make reference to nurses' need to exercise critical judgment in assessing their ability to deliver competent and safe patient care.[85]

Why is there such interest in nurse/patient ratios?

It is not only the duration of a nursing shift and the ability of nurses to accept or decline additional hours that elicit heated discussion from opposing points of view. So too does the question of how many patients a single RN can adequately care for on that shift. The same issues of quality, patient safety, and worker safety are raised in a discussion of nurses' workload, and the idea of having the size and distribution of the hospital's nursing staff dictated strictly by the volume of patients has the potential to cause numerous logistical and recruitment problems. A 2003 study commissioned by AFT

Healthcare, the health care arm of the American Federation of Teachers union, found that while the average medical/surgical RN was caring for eight patients per shift, 83 percent of the respondents to the survey thought that the average patient load should be six or fewer patients per RN per shift.[86]

Whenever the issue of nurse/patient ratios is raised, all eyes turn to California, the first state to legislatively mandate nurse/patient ratios in its hospitals. Signed into law in 1999, the ratio was set at six patients per nurse, effective January 1, 2005. In November 2004 Governor Arnold Schwarzenegger proposed emergency regulations–citing an inadequate supply of nurses to implement the statute–to delay implementation until January 2008. The California Nurses Association, acting on behalf of its union members, sued the governor for acting illegally to delay the law, and in early June 2005 a Sacramento County Superior Court judge handed down a permanent injunction in favor of the nurses,[87] ending a legal battle that had been accompanied by massive public demonstrations organized by nurses around the state.

Whether nurse/patient ratios can be implemented and maintained, whether the ratio set by California law is a standard that can be applied equally across the country, and whether the same ratio should be applied across all types of hospitals remains to be seen. As California sets itself to implement its new nursing model, everyone with a vested interest in health care delivery will be awaiting the results.

What are the turnover and vacancy rates for hospital RNs?

Turnover and vacancy rates vary from survey to survey. A survey of hospital leaders conducted by the AHA in 2004 indicated an RN vacancy rate of 8.4 percent in 2003.[88] An online survey of health care recruiters conducted by the Bernard Hodes Group in late 2004 yielded a 2004 vacancy rate of 16.1 percent.[89] Despite the difference of almost 100 percent between the two percentages quoted, both surveys identified RNs as the employee category with the highest vacancy rate.

Turnover, expressed as a percentage, is the number of positions needing to be filled, divided by all positions in a given time period. The Bernard Hodes survey indicated that RN turnover in 2004 was 13.9 percent, slightly higher than the overall turnover rate of 13.7 percent, but less than for occupational therapists, who logged the highest rate, 14.9 percent.[90] An earlier 2004 survey from

the Hospital & Healthcare Compensation Service reported an RN turnover rate of approximately 14.8 percent.[91]

The costs of high vacancy and turnover rates can be considerable, not only in terms of the impact on staff morale, the continuity and quality of patient care, and patient satisfaction, but also in terms of recruitment and training costs, and the need to devote more and more staff resources to these functions. The Bernard Hodes survey data showed that the average cost per hire for nurses ran just over $2,800; only pharmacist recruitment generated more expenses.[92] A study by Cheryl Bland Jones published in two parts in *JONA: The Journal of Nursing Administration* outlined a tool for assessing nurse turnover costs, the Nursing Turnover Cost Calculation Methodology (NTCCM).[93] Grounded in human capital theory and factoring in pre-hire costs (costs incurred by advertising and recruiting, costs of having vacant positions, and costs of hiring) and post-hire costs (costs of orientation and training, costs of fluctuations in productivity of newly arrived and ready-to-depart nurses, and costs of termination), an application of the NTCCM to a large hospital (600+ beds) revealed turnover costs of 1.2 to 1.3 times RN salary.

What role do foreign nurses play?

The recruitment of nursing professionals from other countries has been used as a strategy for plugging hospitals' staffing gaps for as long as nursing shortages have plagued the health care delivery system. The 2000 National Sample Survey of Registered Nurses from the U.S. Bureau of Health Professions indicated that a little less than 100,000 RNs (approximately 4 percent) received their basic nursing education outside the United States.[94] Although the percentage of the total RN workforce represented by foreign nurses has not exceeded 5 percent historically, the proportion is steadily rising.[95]

The Philippines has been the largest supplier of nurses,[96] at one point representing the country of origin for 75 percent of all foreign nurses in the U.S. RN workforce. That percentage has declined with the influx of nationals from other countries, including India, Nigeria, the United Kingdom, and Canada. Regardless of nationality, all foreign-trained nurses must successfully complete the Commission on Graduates of Foreign Nursing School three-part certification program, Visa Screen–a review of the candidate's education, registration, and licensure credentials; a qualifying exam that tests nursing knowledge; and an English-language proficiency exam—before sitting for a state licensing exam.

The influx of foreign nurses is regulated by the visa requirements and annual quotas established by the U.S. Citizenship and Immigration Services (CIS, formerly Immigration and Naturalization Services), a bureau within the U.S. Department of Homeland Security. Foreign nurses may be eligible for one of several different classes of visas, depending on their country of origin, educational background, and where they wish to work. For example, registered nurses from Canada and Mexico may apply for TN visas, a visa category created under the North American Free Trade Agreement. Nurses with additional responsibilities or training, such as charge nurses, unit supervisors, or advanced practice nurses may be eligible for the H-1B visa. Visas may be temporary (usually issued for a three-year period) or permanent. Hospitals won a major legislative victory in the spring of 2005 when Congress passed a Department of Defense supplemental appropriations bill that reallocated 50,000 unused visas from countries that had not filled them in the past four years to the Philippines, India, and China—three major supply sources of foreign nurses that had exhausted their quota of visas.[97]

As the potential employer, the hospital has the responsibility for initiating the visa process, providing adequate proof that there is a shortage of U.S. workers qualified or willing to fill the vacant positions for which foreign nurses are being recruited, and that the employment of foreign nationals will not adversely affect the wage and working conditions in the United States. It should be noted that recruiting foreign nurses is not a cost-saving measure: The nurses must be paid the prevailing wages for the positions they fill, and there are significant costs associated with the visa application process itself, including application fees, testing fees, legal fees, and any relocation costs the hospital chooses to underwrite. One immigration law expert estimated the ballpark costs of successfully recruiting a foreign nurse at $6,000 to $25,000, depending on whether one includes only direct out-of-pocket expenses or all costs incurred from the initiation of the visa application to the integration of the newly arrived nurse into the hospital's employee pool.[98]

The diversity represented by foreign nurses must be accounted for and accommodated by the organizational cultures of the hospitals and other facilities in which these nurses find employment. Often, foreign-trained nurses are accompanied by their families, for whom adequate housing must be found. On-the-job training must allow for orientation to technologies available only in the United States and the complex protocols of care and documentation that frame every patient encounter.

How has the nursing scope of practice changed?

In the United States, the Civil War is often regarded as the tipping point for nursing as a professional occupation, although in the early stages of the war, nursing was as much about finding food and shelter for the ill and wounded as it was about providing first aid and medical care. However, as the war dragged on, and the nurses, many of them women, proved themselves in hastily improvised battlefield surgeries and field hospitals, their duties became more demanding.[99] Nurse anesthetists mark the origins of their area of practice as a nursing specialty from this time period, and many of the nursing schools that were established in various hospitals in the decades after the war were founded by women who had first seen service in Union or Confederate army hospitals. Nursing as a profession began to evolve, dominated by women dedicated to the vision of Florence Nightingale, Clara Barton, Dorothea Dix, and other nursing pioneers, women who laid the groundwork for nursing theory as well as nursing education.

Professional nursing has kept pace with the developments in medical knowledge and technology. It has adapted to and thrived in every conceivable health care delivery scenario, and the nurse is established as an indispensable member of the patient care team. With the advent of advanced practice nurses, the lines differentiating the professional activities, responsibilities, and privileges of physicians and nurses have not so much blurred as thinned.

Nurses have also moved from the bedside to the boardroom, expanding their role beyond caregiving to strategic planning, IT consultation, and executive management. The 2000 National Sample Survey of Registered Nurses indicated that the dominant function of 4 percent of hospital-employed RNs was administration.[100] An estimated 700 hospital chief executive officers and 540 chief operating officers started their health careers as nurses.[101]

Other Health Professionals

What are some of the other types of important health professionals?

Although physicians and nurses may be the most visible and numerous professional members of the health care team, they are not the only members. The U.S. Bureau of Labor Statistics lists 39 occupations—in addition to the nurse, physician, and veterinary medical occupations—in the category "Healthcare Practitioners and Technical Occupations," including pharmacists, dietitians, nutritionists, physical therapists, radiation therapists, medical/clinical laboratory technicians and technologists, emergency medical technicians and paramedics, and surgical technologists, among others. Of the 6.3 million individuals classified as nonveterinary health care professionals, approximately 2.5 million (40 percent) are in the allied health professions,[102] usually considered to be those health occupations outside of medicine, nursing, dentistry, and podiatry that require special education and/or training.[103] For many allied health professions, certification and/or licensure is also a requirement. The 2004–2005 edition of the American Medical Association's *Health Professions Career and Education Directory* includes 64 occupations, with over 6,500 education and training programs in over 2,400 sponsoring institutions.[104]

Continuing advances in the science, technology, and delivery of health care virtually ensure that no single practitioner or profession can master the field and single-handedly deliver a complete package of care. The skills needed to work with sophisticated imaging equipment in the radiology department are far different from the skills needed to execute the complex diagnostic tests taking place in the clinical laboratory, and different still from the bedside care being provided by RNs and their support staff. Allied health professionals, as part of the hospital-wide patient care team, not only bring to the table specialized knowledge and skills that may not be available from other members of the team, but they also provide a level of flexibility that allows each member of the team to concentrate on delivering the highest level of care his or her own particular training permits.

Is there a shortage of these personnel?

The U.S. workforce shortage has affected not only the pool of available physicians and RNs, but allied health personnel as well. The 2004 AHA Survey of Hospital Leaders indicated that while nursing registered the highest vacancy rate, pharmacists, imaging technicians, and laboratory technicians were also in short supply.[105] The Bernard Hodes Group's *Health Care Metrics Study* identified four categories of therapists (occupational, speech/language, physical, and respiratory) with higher turnovers than RNs, in addition to radiology technicians, pharmacists, and laboratory technicians, with double-digit turnover rates. The same occupations had vacancy rates over 10 percent.[106]

What career opportunities are available?

The following are examples of the careers available in the allied health professions:[107]

Art therapist	Music therapist
Audiologist	Nuclear medicine technologist
Cardiovascular technologist	Occupational therapist
Clinical laboratory technician	Physical therapist
Cytotechnologist	Physician assistant
Diagnostic medical sonographer	Radiation therapist
Dietitian	Radiologic technologist
Electroneurodiagnostic technologist	Rehabilitation counselor
Emergency medical technician	Respiratory therapist
Genetic counselor	Speech/language pathologist
Health information manager	Surgical technologist

Besides offering specialized curricula as a prerequisite for professional practice, many of these occupations also support professional societies that provide practice guidelines and codes of professional conduct, continuing education opportunities, and advocacy at the national, state, and local levels for the profession and the issues that impact it.

Invisible Caregivers

What is the role of family and friends in delivering health care?

As vast as the U.S. health care delivery system is, it is dwarfed both in size and in the number of lives affected by an informal, highly unstructured delivery system composed of family, friends, "significant others," and good Samaritans who provide health care services to people in need at home on an unpaid basis. Existing completely outside of and, in many instances, only remotely connected to the more formal venues of health care delivery, these "invisible" caregivers include an estimated 44.4 million Americans 18 years of age or older– roughly 21 percent of the adult U.S. population. Two-thirds of these caregivers are women, and a little more than half are less than 50 years old. Roughly 48 percent of this group are actively engaged in caregiving activities eight hours a week or less, but almost 17 percent put in 40-plus hours of caregiving duties per week.[108]

Most caregiving recipients are older adults: 79 percent are at least 50 years old, and 20 percent are 80 years of age or older. The most prevalent health problems of these individuals simply involve the effects of old age; however, cancer, diabetes, heart disease, Alzheimer's disease or other dementia, stroke, arthritis, and blindness or limited vision are also common. Formal diagnosis is difficult, but it is estimated that 23 percent of recipients suffer from Alzheimer's or some other form of dementia. Of the caregiver recipients who are younger than 50, the most prevalent health condition (affecting 23 percent) is mental illness.[109]

Transportation is the primary "lifestyle" need presented by caregiving recipients, and 82 percent of caregivers provide this service. Grocery shopping (75 percent), housekeeping duties (69 percent), finance management (64 percent), and meal preparation (59 percent) are the other services most often provided. Forty-one percent of caregivers assist with or manage the recipient's medication. Caregivers also provide more personal care: assistance with getting into and out of bed/chair (36 percent), dressing (29 percent), bathing/showering (26 percent), getting to/from the toilet (23 percent), eating (18 percent), and dealing with incontinence (16 percent).[110] The average duration of caregiving is a little over four years, although almost a third of caregivers actively provide care for five years or more.[111]

How does this role intersect with the health care system?

Forty percent of caregivers use paid care at least once a year to supplement their own, more informal services. This solicitation of support runs the gamut from engaging the services of a home health nurse to hiring a housekeeper.[112] Even taking into account some level of reliance on the more formal channels of health care delivery, a conservative estimate of the annual value of the informal caregiving provided by family and friends is $257 billion.[113] It is inconceivable that this amount of care could be provided by a delivery system already strapped for personnel, resources, and funding.

The National Alliance for Caregiving, a coalition of over forty national organizations (including AARP, the National Council on Aging, and the U.S. Department of Veterans Affairs), has positioned itself as an advocate for the invisible caregivers and has promulgated a set of principles designed to formally acknowledge both the contributions and needs of caregivers and to carve a place for them in U.S. health care and social policy.[114] Since 1996 the United Hospital Fund of New York City has been supporting research, disseminating findings, and funding grants through its Families and Health Care Project.[115]

For their part, hospitals must make a conscious effort to involve caregivers in the patient care team and recognize that, although not sharing the scientific and technical expertise of the formally trained team members, the caregiver is usually *the* expert on the patient, intimately acquainted with the patient's life and medical history and, more often than not, responsible for the care the patient will receive following discharge from the hospital.

References

1. Felix Barber and Rainer Strack, "The Surprising Economics of a 'People Business,'" *Harvard Business Review* 83, no. 6 (June 2005): 80–90.
2. U.S. Department of Labor, Bureau of Labor Statistics, *Employment, Hours, and Earnings from the Current Employment Statistics Survey (National)*, Series CES0000000001 and CES6562000101, http://data.bls.gov/cgi-bin/srgate (data extracted March 2005).
3. U.S. Department of Labor, *Employment, Hours, and Earnings*, Series ID CES6562200001, http://data.bls.gov/cgi-bin/srgate (data extracted March 2005).
4. American Hospital Association, "State-by-State Analysis Highlights Hospitals' Impact on Communities" (Press Release, May 3, 2004), http://www.aha.org/aha/press_room-info/jsp/releasedisplay.jsp?dcrpath=AHA/Press_Release/data/PR_040503_StateByState&domain=AHA (accessed June 21, 2005).
5. American Hospital Association, *Hospital Statistics*, 2005 ed. (Chicago: Health Forum, 2005): 7.
6. Gerald A. Doeksen, Tom Johnson, and Chuck Willoughby, *Measuring the Economic Importance of the*

Health Sector on a Local Economy: A Brief Literature Review and Procedures to Measure Local Impacts (Mississippi State: Southern Rural Development Center, 1997), http://srdc.msstate.edu/publications/202.pdf (accessed June 27, 2005); Sam Cordes, Evert Vander Sluis, Charles Lampher, and Jerry Hoffman, "Rural Hospitals and the Local Economy: A Needed Extension and Refinement of Existing Empirical Research," *Journal of Rural Health* 15, no. 2 (Spring 1999): 189–201.

7. Peter F. Drucker, *Management: Tasks, Responsibilities, Practices* (New York: Harper & Row, 1974): 4.

8. U.S. Department of Labor, Bureau of Labor Statistics, *November 2003 National Industry-Specific Occupational Employment and Wage Estimates: NAICS 622000-Hospitals,* http://www.bls.gov/oes/current/naics3_622000.htm#b00-0000 (accessed June 21, 2005).

9. B. Jon Jaeger, ed., *Revisiting the Three-Legged Stool: Striking a New Balance Among Trustees, Administrators, and Physicians. Report of the 1990 National Forum on Hospital and Health Affairs.* (Durham, NC: Duke University, Department of Health Administration, 1991): v.

10. Institute of Medicine, Committee on Quality of Health Care in America, *Crossing the Quality Chasm: A New Health System for the 21st Century.* (Washington, DC: National Academy Press, 2001): 83.

11. Shari Mycek, "Getting to Know You: An Open Dialogue Between the Board and Physicians Will Jump-Start Better Relations," *Trustee* 57, no. 4 (April 2004): 22–25.

12. AHA Commission on Workforce for Hospitals and Health Systems, *In Our Hands: How Hospital Leaders Can Build a Thriving Workforce* (Chicago: American Hospital Association, 2002): 7–8.

13. Richard C. McKibbin and Carol Boston, *The Nursing Shortage: Opportunities and Solutions. Monograph 1: An Overview: Characteristics, Impact and Solutions* (Chicago: American Organization of Nurse Executives, 1990): 2.

14. Michael R. Bleich and Peggy O. Hewlett, "Dissipating the 'Perfect Storm'—Responses from Nursing and the Health Care Industry to Protect the Public's Health," *Online Journal of Issues in Nursing* 9, no. 2, ms. no. 4 (May 31, 2004), http://www.nursingworld.org/ojin/topic24/tpc24_4.htm (accessed June 27, 2005).

15. Bernard Hodes Group, *Health Care Metrics Study* (New York: Bernard Hodes Group, 2004): 10, http://www.hodes.com/healthcarematters/pdfs/HodesHCMetricsReport_2004.PDF (accessed March 18, 2005).

16. Ann E. Rogers, Wei-Ting Hwang, Linda D. Scott, Linda H. Aiken, and David F. Dinges, "The Working Hours of Hospital Staff Nurses and Patient Safety," *Health Affairs* 23, no. 4 (July/August 2004): 202–212, http://content.healthaffairs.org/cgi/reprint/23/4/202 (accessed June 28, 2005).

17. Juliana M. Sadovich, "Work Excitement in Nursing: An Examination of the Relationship Between Work Excitement and Burnout," *Nursing Economics* 23, no. 2 (March–April 2005): 91–96.

18. AHA Commission on Workforce, *In Our Hands.* (Subsequent reports, titled *Workforce Ideas in Action: Case Examples,* were issued in January and September 2003, and January and June 2004. Extracts from these publications, as well as a variety of tools, calendars of educational events, and other relevant sources of information can be found at http://www.healthcareworkforce.org/healthcareworkforce/index.jsp.

19. Ernell Spratley, Ayah Johnson, Julie Sochalski, Marshall Fritz, and William Spencer, *The Registered Nurse Population, March 2000: Findings from the National Sample of Registered Nurses.* (Washington, DC: U.S. Department of Health and Human Services, Health Resources and Services Administration, Bureau of Health Professions, Division of Nursing, 2002): 8–11, ftp://ftp.hrsa.gov/bhpr/rnsurvey2000/rnsurvey00.pdf (accessed April 1, 2005).

20. Sarah Dore, "2004 Rate Survey Indicates Rate Increases May Be Leveling But Triple-Digit Hikes Not Over," *Medical Liability Monitor* 29, no. 10 (October 2004): 1–5.

21. Catherine Thomas, ed., *Current Award Trends in Personal Injury,* 44th ed. (Horsham, PA: LRP Publications, 2005): 22.

22. Dore, "2004 Rate Survey."

23. Ron Shinkman, "The Disappearing Doctor: What's the Status of Liability Insurance in Your State?" *Trustee* 58, no. 6 (June 2005): 6–10. The article includes a sidebar listing 20 states identified by the American Medical Association as experiencing a "severe medical malpractice liability insurance crisis." These states are Arkansas, Connecticut, Florida, Georgia, Illinois, Kentucky, Massachusetts, Mississippi, Missouri, Nevada, New Jersey, New York, North Carolina, Ohio, Oregon, Pennsylvania, Texas, Washington, West Virginia, and Wyoming.

24. Thomas Pasko and Derek R. Smart, *Physician Characteristics and Distribution in the U.S.,* 2005 ed. (Chicago: American Medical Association, 2005): 8.

25. American Osteopathic Association, *About the AOA,* http://www.osteopathic.org/index.cfm?PageID=aoa_main (accessed April 15, 2005).

26. Douglas M. Anderson, Jeff Keith, Patricia D. Novak, and Michelle A. Elliot, *Mosby's Medical, Nursing, & Allied Health Dictionary,* 6th ed. (St. Louis, MO: Mosby, 2002): 67

27. American Osteopathic Association, *OMT: Hands-On Care,* http://www.osteopathic.org/index.cfm?PageID=ost_omt (accessed April 15, 2005).

28. U.S. Department of Health and Human Services, Health Resources and Services Administration, Council on Graduate Medical Education, *Physician Workforce Policy Guidelines for the United States, 2000–2020* (Washington, DC: U.S. Department of Health and Human Services, January 2005): xvi.

29. U.S. Department of Health and Human Services, Public Health Service, Health Resources Administration, Office of Graduate Medical Education, Graduate Medical Education Advisory Committee, *Report of the Graduate Medical Education National Advisory Committee to the Secretary, Department of Health and Human Services* (Washington, DC: U.S. Department of Health and Human Services, 1981).

30. H.J. Simmons III and John M. Harris, "Market Memo: Community-Based Physician Need Planning Methodologies Evolve," *Health Care Strategic Management* 22, no. 12 (December 2004): 1, 14–19.

31. U.S. Department of Health and Human Services, Health Resources and Services Administration, Bureau of Health Professions, *Shortage Designation*, http://bhpr.hrsa.gov/shortage/ (accessed April 15, 2005).

32. American Board of Medical Specialties, *ABMS Member Boards: General Certificates Issued, 1994–2003*, http://www.abms.org/Downloads/ Statistics/Table2.PDF; American Board of Medical Specialties, *ABMS Member Boards: Subspecialty Certificates Issued, 1994–2003*, http://www.abms.org/ Downloads/Statistics/Table4.PDF (accessed April 15, 2005).

33. Pasko and Smart, *Physician Characteristics*: 335–337.

34. Ibid.: 9.

35. Jack M. Colwill and James M. Cultice, "The Future Supply of Family Physicians: Implications for Rural America," *Health Affairs* 22, no. 1 (January–February 2003): 190–198, http://content.healthaffairs.org/cgi/reprint/22/1/190 (accessed June 15, 2005).

36. Barbara Starfield, Leiyu Shi, Atul Grover, and James Macinko, "The Effects of Specialist Supply on Populations' Health: Assessing the Evidence," *Health Affairs* (March 15, 2005): W5-97–107, http://content.healthaffairs.org/cgi/reprint/ hlthaff.w5.97v1 (accessed June 15, 2005).

37. U.S. Department of Health and Human Services, Centers for Disease Control and Prevention, National Center for Health Statistics, *Health, United States, 2004: With Chartbook on Trends in the Health of Americans* (Hyattsville, MD: U.S. National Center for Health Statistics, September 2004): 277–279, http://www.cdc.gov/nchs/data/hus/ hus04trend.pdf#topic (accessed June 15, 2005).

38. National Library of Medicine, *Changing the Face of Medicine: Dr. Elizabeth Blackwell*, http://www.nlm.nih.gov/changingthefaceofmedicine/ physicians/biography_35.html (accessed April 27, 2005); National Library of Medicine, *Changing the Face of Medicine: Dr. Emily Blackwell*, http://www.nlm.nih.gov/changingthefaceofmedicine/ physicians/biography_36.html (accessed April 27, 2005).

39. Pasko and Smart, *Physician Characteristics*: 8; Phillip R. Kletke, William D. Marder, and Anne B. Silberger, "The Growing Proportion of Female Physicians: Implications for U.S. Physician Supply," *American Journal of Public Health* 80, no. 3 (March 1990): 300–304.

40. Julia E. McMurray, Graham Angus, May Cohen, Paul Gavel, John Harding, John Horvath, Elisabeth Paice, Julie Schmittdiel, and Kevin Grumbach, "Women in Medicine: A Four-Nation Comparison," *Journal of the American Medical Women's Association* 57, no. 4 (Fall 2002): 185–190.

41. Debra L. Roter, Judith A. Hall, and Yutaka Aoki, "Physician Gender Effects in Medical Communication: A Meta-analytic Review," *JAMA* 288, no. 6 (August 14, 2002): 756–764.

42. Klea D. Bertakis, Peter Franks, and Rahman Azari, "Effects of Physician Gender on Patient Satisfaction," *Journal of the American Medical Women's Association* 58, no. 2 (Spring 2003): 69–75.

43. Arlene S. Ash, Phyllis L. Carr, Richard Goldstein, and Robert H. Friedman, "Compensation and Advancement of Women in Academic Medicine: Is There Equity?" *Annals of Internal Medicine* 141, no. 3 (August 3, 2004): 205–212, W43–44.

44. LeEtta Robinson, ed., *AAMC Data Book: Statistical Information Related to Medical Schools and Teaching Hospitals* (Washington, DC: Association of American Medical Colleges, 2003): 22.

45. U.S. Census Bureau, *Projected Population of the United States, by Race and Hispanic Origin: 2000–2050* (March 18, 2004), http://www.census.gov/ ipc/www/usinterimproj/natprojtab01a.xls (accessed May 6, 2005).

46. American College of Physicians, "Racial and Ethnic Disparities in Health Care: A Position Paper of the American College of Physicians," *Annals of Internal Medicine* 141, no. 3 (August 3, 2004): 226–232, http://www.acponline.org/hpp/healthcare_disp.pdf (accessed June 23, 2005).

47. Neil R. Powe and Lisa A. Cooper, "Diversifying the Racial and Ethnic Composition of the Physician Workforce," *Annals of Internal Medicine* 141, no. 3 (August 3, 2004): 223–224.

48. Rick Pollack, Executive Vice President, American Hospital Association, letter to the Honorable Ralph Regula, Chairman, House Appropriations Subcommittee, Labor, Health and Human Services and Education (April 28, 2004), http://www.aha.org/ aha/advocacy-grassroots/advocacy/hillletters/ content/042804Hillet_appropriate.doc (accessed May 9, 2005).

49. Lawton R. Burns, "Physician Practice Management Companies," *Health Care Management Review* 22, no. 4 (Fall 1997): 32–46, http://hcmg.wharton.upenn.edu/burnsl/PDF%20Files/Physician%20Practice%20-%20HCMG%20Review.pdf (accessed April 27, 2005).

50. Stephen Kraft, "Physician Practice Management Companies: A Failed Concept," *Physician Executive* 28, no. 2 (March–April 2002): 54–57, http://www.findarticles.com/p/articles/mi_m0843/is_2_28/ai_84236566/print (accessed April 27, 2005); Uwe E. Reinhardt, "The Rise and Fall of the Physician Practice Management Industry," *Health Affairs* 19, no. 1 (January–February 2000): 42–55, http://content.healthaffairs.org/cgi/reprint/19/1/42 (accessed April 27, 2005); Tom Nash, "Physician Practice Management Companies: What Went Wrong and Where Do We Go from Here?" *Jacksonville Medicine* (February 1999), http://www.dcmsonline.org/jax-medicine/1999journals/february99/practice.htm (accessed April 27, 2005).

51. Verispan, *2003 Guide to Healthcare Market Segments* (Chicago: Verispan, 2003): 126.

52. Justin C. Matus, "Boutique Medicine: Good Medicine with a Bad Taste or Just Bad Medicine?" *AAMA Executive* (Winter 2003), http://www.aameda.org/MemberServices/Exec/Articles/winter03/boutiquemedMatus.pdf (accessed June 28, 2005).

53. American College of Surgeons, Committee on Trauma, *Resources for Optimal Care of the Injured Patient: 1999* (Chicago: ACS, 1998): 10–11; American Academy of Pediatrics and the American College of Obstetricians and Gynecologists, *Guidelines for Perinatal Care*, 5th ed. (Elk Grove Village, IL: AAP; Washington, DC: ACOG, 2002): 17–21.

54. Richard Haugh, "Are You Looking for a Fresh Start with Your MDs?" *Hospitals & Health Networks* 79, no. 5 (May 2005): 36–38, 40, 42.

55. The Governance Institute, *Governance Forecast: Board Performance, Challenges, & Opportunities* (San Diego, CA: TGI, 2003): 5–6.

56. American Hospital Association. *Protecting the Health Care Safety Net: Limited Service Hospitals* (Washington, DC: American Hospital Association, 2005), http://www.aha.org/aha/annual_meeting/content/05_limitedservhosp.pdf (accessed September 28, 2005).

57. David A. Woodwell and Donald K. Cherry, "National Ambulatory Medical Care Survey: 2002 Summary," *Advance Data* no. 346 (August 26, 2004): 1–44, http://www.cdc.gov/nchs/data/ad/ad346.pdf (accessed June 27, 2005).

58. Society of Hospital Medicine, *Definition of a Hospitalist* (2005), http://www.hospitalmedicine.org/Content/NavigationMenu/AboutSHM/DefinitionofaHospitalist/Definition_of_a_Hosp.htm (accessed May 14, 2005).

59. Robert M. Wachter and Lee Goldman, "The Emerging Role of 'Hospitalists' in the American Health Care System," *New England Journal of Medicine* 335, no. 7 (August 15, 1996): 514–517; Maureen Glabman, "Hospitalists: The Next Big Thing?" *Trustee* 58, no. 5 (May 2005): 6–11.

60. Dagmara Scalise, "Around the Clock Care: With Hospitalists on Board, Patients Get 24-Hour Physician Attention," *Hospitals & Health Networks* 79, no. 5 (May 2005): 20, 22.

61. Glabman, "Hospitalists"

62. Christopher J. Gearon, "Medicine's Turf Wars: Specialists Without M.D.'s Are Pushing for More Medical Power. Are They Ready–And Are You?" *U.S. News & World Report* 138, no. 4 (January 1, 2005), http://www.usnews.com/usnews/health/articles/05131/31turf.htm (accessed June 2, 2005).

63. Mary P. Malone, Executive Director of Consulting Services, Press Ganey Associates, quoted in Laurie Larson, "Restoring the Relationship: The Key to Nurse and Patient Satisfaction," *Trustee* 57, no. 9 (October 2004): 8–10, 12, 14.

64. Anderson, *Mosby's Medical, Nursing, & Allied Health Dictionary*: 1479.

65. U.S. Department of Labor, Bureau of Labor Statistics, *Occupational Employment and Wages, May 2004: 29-1111 Registered Nurses* (June 2, 2005), http://www.bls.gov/oes/current/oes291111.htm (accessed June 4, 2005).

66. American Nurses Association, *About the American Nurses Association* (2005), http://nursingworld.org/about/ (accessed June 5, 2005).

67. U.S. Department of Labor, *Occupational Employment and Wages*.

68. Aaron Dalton, "All for One: Through a Joint Marketing Campaign, Hospitals Hope to Lure Workers to Their City," *Hospitals & Health Networks* 78, no. 12 (December 2004): 22, 24, http://www.hhnmag.com/hhnmag/hospitalconnect/search/article.jsp?dcrpath=HHNMAG/PubsNewsArticle/data/0412HHN_InBox_Workforce&domain=HHNMAG (accessed June 4, 2005).

69. AHA Commission on Workforce, *In Our Hands*: 65–70.

70. Margaret L. McClure, Muriel A. Poulin, Margaret D. Sovie, and Mabel A. Wandelt, *Magnet Hospitals: Attraction and Retention of Professional Nurses* (Kansas City, MO: American Nurses Association, 1983).

71. Margaret L. McClure and Ada Sue Hinshaw, *Magnet Hospitals Revisited: Attraction and Retention of Professional Nurses* (Washington, DC: American Nurses Association, 2002): 106–107.

72. American Nurses Credentialing Center, *Magnet Facilities* (June 1, 2005), http://www.nursingworld.org/ancc/magnet/facilities.html (accessed June 4, 2005).

73. American Hospital Association, "Hospital Schools of Nursing," in *American Hospital Association Guide to the Health Care Field*, 1995 ed. (Chicago: AHA, 1995): A489–490; American Hospital Association, "Hospital Schools of Nursing," in *AHA Guide to the Health Care Field*, 2005 ed. (Chicago: Health Forum, 2004): A892.

74. American Association of Colleges of Nursing, "New Data Confirms Shortage of Nursing School Faculty Hinders Efforts to Address the Nation's Nursing Shortage" (Press Release, March 8, 2005), http://www.aacn.nche.edu/Media/NewsReleases/2005/Enrollments05.htm (accessed June 6, 2005).

75. Spratley et al., *Registered Nurse Population*: 19.

76. Ibid.: 20.

77. U.S. Department of Health and Human Services, Health Resources and Services Administration, Bureau of Health Professions, National Center for Health Workforce Analysis, *Projected Supply, Demand, and Shortages of Registered Nurses: 2000–2020* (July 2002): 6, ftp://ftp.hrsa.gov/bhpr/nationalcenter/rnproject.pdf (accessed June 6, 2005).

78. U.S. Department of Health and Human Services, *Projected Supply, Demand, and Shortages*: 7.

79. Jan Greene, "What Nurses Want: Different Generations, Different Expectations," *Hospitals & Health Networks* 79, no. 3 (March 2005): 34–36, 38, 40, 42, http://www.hhnmag.com/hhnmag/hospitalconnect/search/article.jsp?dcrpath=HHNMAG/PubsNewsArticle/data/0503HHN_FEA_CoverStory&domain=HHNMAG (accessed June 6, 2005).

80. American Nurses Association, *Opposition to Mandatory Overtime* (October 17, 2001), http://www.nursingworld.org/readroom/position/workplac/revmot2.htm (accessed June 6, 2005).

81. Rogers et al., "Working Hours of Hospital Staff Nurses."

82. U.S. Department of Labor, Employment Standards Administration, Wage and Hour Division, *Fact Sheet #17N: Nurses and the Part 541 Exemptions Under the Fair Labor Standards Act (FLSA)*, http://www.dol.gov/esa/regs/compliance/whd/fairpay/fs17n_nurses.htm (accessed June 6, 2005).

83. Gina Rollins, "Who's Exempt? New Overtime Rules Still Getting Scrutiny from Nurse Unions and Lawmakers," *Hospitals & Health Networks* 79, no. 4 (April 2005): 30, http://www.hhnmag.com/hhnmag/hospitalconnect/search/article.jsp?dcrpath=HHNMAG/PubsNewsArticle/data/0504HHN_InBox_Workforce1&domain=HHNMAG (accessed June 2, 2005).

84. American Nurses Association, *Staffing Issues: Connecticut Is 10th State to Limit Mandatory Overtime* (May 2004), http://www.nursingworld.org/staffing/ct10th.htm (accessed June 6, 2005).

85. American Nurses Association, *Opposition to Mandatory Overtime*.

86. Peter D. Hart Research Associates, *Patient-to-Nurse Staffing Ratios: Perspectives from Hospital Nurses* (Washington, DC: AFT Healthcare, April 2003): 3, http://www.aft.org/pubs-reports/healthcare/HartStaffingReport2003.pdf (accessed June 11, 2005).

87. "California Judge Issues Final Ruling on Nursing Ratios," *AONE eNews Update* (June 10, 2005), http://www.aone.org/aone/pubs/enews/June%2005/061005.html (accessed June 13, 2005).

88. American Hospital Association, *Overview of the U.S. Health Care System* (February 2005), http://www.aha.org/aha/nhcp/content/Overview.ppt (accessed June 6, 2005).

89. Bernard Hodes Group, *Health Care Metrics Study*: 10.

90. Bernard Hodes Group, *Health Care Metrics Study*: 9.

91. Hospital & Healthcare Compensation Service, *2004–2005 Hospital Salary & Benefits Report* (Oakland, NJ: Hospital & Healthcare Compensation Service, 2004): 15.

92. Bernard Hodes Group, *Health Care Metrics Study*: 11.

93. Cheryl B. Jones, "The Costs of Nurse Turnover, Part 1: An Economic Perspective," *JONA* 34, no. 12 (December 2004): 562–570; Cheryl B. Jones, "The Costs of Nurse Turnover, Part 2: Application of the Nursing Turnover Cost Calculation Methodology," *JONA* 35, no. 1 (January 2005): 41–49.

94. Spratley et al., *Registered Nurse Population*: 33.

95. Barbara L. Brush, Julie Sochalski, and Anne M. Berger, "Imported Care: Recruiting Foreign Nurses to U.S. Health Care Facilities," *Health Affairs* 23, no. 3 (May–June 2004): 78–87, http://content.healthaffairs.org/cgi/reprint/23/3/78 (accessed June 8, 2005).

96. Ibid.: 79; Commission on Graduates of Foreign Nursing Schools, *2004 Annual Report: Global Connections* (Philadelphia: CGFNS, 2005): 15, http://www.cgfns.org/pdf/2004_annual_report.pdf (accessed June 8, 2005).

97. "Congress Reassigns Visas to Help Ease U.S. Nurse Shortage," *AHA News Now* (May 11, 2005), http://www.ahanews.com/ahanews/hospitalconnect/search/article.jsp?dcrpath=AHANEWS/AHANewsNowArticle/data/ann_050511_visa&domain=AHANEWS (accessed June 8, 2005).

98. James Maycock, interviewed in Lisette Hilton, "The Legal Scoop on Hiring International Nurses," *Nursing Spectrum* (November 22, 2004), http://www.helpatnursingspectrum.com/recruiters/load_article.html?AID=897 (accessed October 9, 2005).

99. Victoria L. Holder, "From Hand Maiden to Right Hand–The Birth of Nursing in America," *AORN Journal* 78, no. 4 (October 2003): 618–632.

100. Spratley et al., *Registered Nurse Population*: 23.
101. Patrick Reilly, "Front Lines to Front Office," *Modern Healthcare* 34, no. 16 (April 19, 2004): 24, 26, 28.
102. U.S. Department of Labor, Bureau of Labor Statistics, *May 2004 National Occupational Employment and Wage Estimates: Healthcare Practitioner and Technical Occupations* (June 2, 2005), http://www.bls.gov/oes/current/oes_29he.htm (accessed June 11, 2005).
103. Anderson, *Mosby's Medical, Nursing & Allied Health Dictionary*: 1278.
104. American Medical Association, *Health Professions Career and Education Directory, 2004–2005*, 32nd ed. (Chicago: AMA, 2004): vi.
105. American Hospital Association, *Overview of the U.S. Health Care System*.
106. Bernard Hodes Group, *Health Care Metrics Study*: 9–10.
107. American Medical Association, *Health Professions Career and Education Directory*: iii–iv.
108. National Alliance for Caregiving and American Association of Retired Persons, *Caregiving in the U.S.* (Bethesda, MD: NAC; Washington, DC: AARP, 2005): vi, http://www.caregiving.org/data/04execsumm.pdf (accessed June 11, 2005).
109. National Alliance for Caregiving, *Caregiving in the U.S.*: 10–11.
110. Ibid.: 14–15.
111. Ibid.: 7.
112. Ibid.: 16–17.
113. P.S. Arno, *Economic Value of Informal Caregiving*, paper presented at Orlando, Florida, Annual Meeting of the American Association of Geriatric Psychiatry, February 2004, cited in Lynn F. Feinberg, Jane Horvath, Gail Hunt, Les Plooster, Jill Kagan, Carol Levine, Joanne Lynn, Suzanne Mintz, and Ann Wilkinson, *Family Caregiving and Public Policy: Principles for Change* (Bethesda, MD: National Alliance for Caregiving, 2003), http://www.caregiving.org/data/principles04.pdf (accessed June 11, 2005).
114. Feinberg, *Family Caregiving*.
115. United Hospital Fund of New York City, *Project Background* (New York: UHFNCY, 2005), http://www.uhfnyc.org/homepage3219/homepage_show.htm?doc_id=103742 (accessed June 11, 2005).

This bill . . . lays a groundwork for providing more and better medical care for the people of our country. Its aim is to assist states in the construction of necessary physical facilities for furnishing adequate hospital, clinical and similar services to all their people.

(Harry S Truman, August 13, 1946)

In the summer of 1946, President Harry Truman signed the landmark Hospital Survey and Construction Act. More commonly known as the Hill-Burton Act, the new law authorized funding for the modernization of existing hospitals and the construction of new hospitals across the country, providing a welcome infusion of capital after the Great Depression and war years. The Hill-Burton program authorized about $1 billion for the first 5 years.[1] Like the postwar years, the nation is again in a health care building boom. But today, a major building project *for a single hospital* can cost hundreds of millions of dollars.

Although the delivery of health care is essentially a person-to-person interaction, the bricks-and-mortar of health care facilities house the high-tech equipment and support staff needed to deliver care efficiently. These facilities range from the solo practitioner's office to the academic medical center. The various types of inpatient and outpatient health care facilities will be described in this chapter.

Hospitals

The effect of the Hill-Burton Act in spurring growth in the number of hospitals after 1946 can be seen in table 3–1. All types of hospitals are included in this count. The total number of hospitals increased from about 6,100 in 1946, peaked at about 7,100 in the mid-1970s, and then decreased to the nearly 5,800 registered hospitals in operation today.

Among the reasons for the decrease in the number of U.S. hospitals after the early 1980s are changes in reimbursement and in medical technology. The old cost-based reimbursement system for Medicare inpatient services was replaced by a prospective payment system. The new system established a predetermined payment rate per discharge and introduced a powerful incentive to shorten the number of days that Medicare patients are hospitalized. At the same time, managed care plans were increasing in influence and establishing their own incentives to curb inpatient utilization. These cost-cutting initiatives were aided by advances in medical technology that contributed not only to shortening hospital inpatient stays but also to shifting care to

Table 3–1. Number of U.S. Registered Hospitals

Year	Number of Hospitals
1946	6,125
1950	6,788
1960	6,876
1970	7,123
1980	6,965
1990	6,649
2000	5,810
2004	5,759

Source: AHA Hospital Statistics, 2006 ed. (Chicago: Health Forum, 2006): 2.

the outpatient setting. As a result of these environmental changes, some hospitals were closed and others were consolidated.[2]

Looking Back at Our Roots
What were the early hospitals like?
In colonial days, the sick and homeless were cared for in government-supported almshouses. Community leaders and physicians, however, believed that there should be a separate charity institution dedicated to healing the sick and injured. Pennsylvania Hospital, founded in Philadelphia in 1751 by Benjamin Franklin and Dr. Thomas Bond, became the nation's first hospital, followed by The New York Hospital and Boston's Massachusetts General Hospital.

Many people preferred to stay at home and receive care there because infection and death rates were high in hospitals. Patients in charity care were also expected to assist with nursing, laundry, and cleaning. Therefore, the wealthy and middle class preferred to stay home and be attended by physicians making house calls.

Public attitudes toward hospital care began to change as advances in science, such as the theory that germs and bacteria cause infection, and a new emphasis on hospitals' cleanliness and sterile surgical equipment, reduced the risk of death in hospitals. Physicians could provide more effective diagnosis and treatment. Hospitals became training grounds for physicians and nurses. The first nursing school opened in 1872 at the New England Hospital for Women and Children in Boston. Hospitals began to be seen as the center of medicine based on science, with skilled professionals involved in patient care. By the 1920s, the hospital as we know it had emerged.[3]

Community Hospitals
What is a community hospital?
There are many possible ways to describe hospitals: public or private, not-for-profit or investor-owned, general or special, teaching or nonteaching, urban or rural, small or large. The American Hospital Association (AHA) has defined a category that encompasses the majority of hospitals in the United States. The nearly 5,000 hospitals known as *community hospitals* range from small critical-access hospitals to large academic medical centers. These community hospitals share the following characteristics:

- Nonfederal ownership—includes hospitals operated by state or local government as well as private not-for-profit and investor-owned hospitals
- Short-term patients—includes hospitals that discharge the majority of their patients within 30 days
- Service type—includes general hospitals as well as certain types of special hospitals

Examples of hospitals that are not included in the community hospital category are federal hospitals such as Veterans Affairs and military hospitals, long-term hospitals, and some types of special hospitals, such as psychiatric hospitals.

In 2004, there were a total of 5,759 registered hospitals in the United States, of which 4,919 were classified as community hospitals.[4] About 70 percent of U.S. registered community hospitals have 200 beds or fewer, and nearly half have fewer than 100 beds, as shown in figure 3–1.

What is a tertiary care hospital?
Health care is sometimes categorized by the level of care provided, from basic to the most complex subspecialty care. When referring to hospitals, the most commonly used term is tertiary care, which implies that the facility provides specialized diagnostic and treatment services. The term *tertiary care hospital* is loosely defined. However, detailed criteria delineating levels of care have been developed for certain types of hospital services, such as neonatal and trauma care.[5]

What is a center of excellence?
A *center of excellence* is a clinical service line developed to be a market leader, serving to attract referrals and differentiate the hospital from competitors. Cardiology, orthopedics, and women's health are among the specialties often chosen

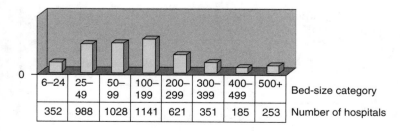

Bed-size category	6–24	25–49	50–99	100–199	200–299	300–399	400–499	500+
Number of hospitals	352	988	1028	1141	621	351	185	253

Figure 3–1. U.S. registered community hospitals by bed size, 2004.

Source: AHA Hospital Statistics, 2006 ed. (Chicago: Health Forum, 2006): 10.

for development as centers of excellence. The Medicare program experimented with centers of excellence during the 1990s, but with a different objective: saving money. Medicare achieved savings of $40 million in a coronary-artery bypass surgery centers of excellence demonstration, which involved a small number of hospitals that had agreed to a bundled hospital-physician payment. An incentive offered to hospitals in this project was the opportunity to market their designation as federally-recognized cardiovascular surgery centers of excellence. Another federal program intended to support the development of centers of excellence is the National Centers of Excellence in Women's Health, which awards the designation and provides grant funding to qualified academic medical centers.[6]

Who owns hospitals?

Some hospitals are owned by federal, state, and local government bodies. The federal government operates more than 200 Veterans Affairs, military, Public Health Service, and other hospitals. States, counties, cities, and local hospital districts operate about five times as many hospitals as the federal government. But the majority of hospitals in the United States are owned and operated by nongovernmental entities, as shown in figure 3–2. Most of these nongovernmental hospitals are owned and operated by not-for-profit secular and religious organizations. Others are owned by investor-owned (for-profit) corporations, such as the large, publicly-traded, multi-institutional systems HCA and Tenet Healthcare Corporation. Investor-owned hospitals also include those owned by partnerships or individuals.

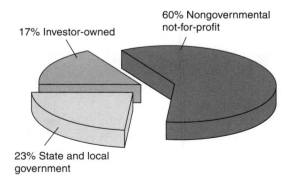

Figure 3–2. U.S. registered community hospitals by ownership, 2004.

Source: AHA Hospital Statistics, 2006 ed. (Chicago: Health Forum, 2006): 6.

What is a critical-access hospital, and how many are there?

Small rural hospitals face many challenges. In an attempt to avert the closure of these vital community resources, Congress authorized a critical-access hospital program as part of the Balanced Budget Act of 1997. The principal advantage of designation as a critical-access hospital is exemption from the Medicare prospective payment system, with the hospital receiving a cost-based payment instead. To be designated as a critical-access hospital, an institution must meet criteria including:

- Location in a rural area at a specified distance from other hospitals
- Provision of emergency services on a 24-hour basis
- Maximum average length of stay of 96 hours

As of early 2005, there were 1,088 critical-access hospitals located in 45 states, representing just under half of all rural hospitals in the country. States with the most critical-access hospitals include Kansas, Iowa, Nebraska, Minnesota, and Texas.[7]

What is a safety-net hospital?

A safety-net hospital is a hospital or health system that provides a significant level of care to low-income, uninsured, and vulnerable populations. Some safety-net hospitals are owned and operated by local or state governments, and others are nongovernmental not-for-profit hospitals. Therefore, rather than being distinguished from other providers by ownership, they are distinguished by their commitment to providing access to health care for people who would otherwise have limited or no access because of financial or insurance status or health condition.[8]

Limited-Service Providers

What is a limited-service provider?

Limited-service providers include hospitals and outpatient facilities that focus on specific conditions or procedures. In some cases, these facilities are part of the continuum of care offered by a full-service community hospital or multi-institutional system. Some are set up as joint ventures between community hospitals and physicians. A recent trend has been the development of limited-service providers owned by physician or corporate entrepreneurs, and it is these facilities that have been the focus of national attention.[9]

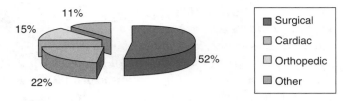

Figure 3–3. Limited-service hospitals by type, 2004.

Source: American Hospital Association, "Impact of Limited-Service Providers on Communities and Full-Service Hospitals," *Trend Watch* 6, no. 2 (September 2004): 1, http://www.ahapolicyforum.org/ahapolicyforum/trendwatch/content/040924_twvol6no2limitedserv.pdf (accessed June 28, 2005).

In 2003, there were an estimated 113 limited-service hospitals in operation with some 30 more under development. Many of these new hospitals have opened within the previous decade. The most common types of limited-service hospitals are surgical hospitals, heart hospitals, and orthopedic hospitals, as seen in figure 3–3.[10]

Do these limited-service hospitals compete with community hospitals?

Limited-service hospitals compete with community hospitals for market share in well-reimbursed service lines. Losing patient volume in these service lines drains resources from full-service community hospitals that rely on this reimbursement to cross-subsidize other essential community services, such as emergency departments.[11]

Concerns about the potential detrimental effect of this competitive situation have prompted several major studies mandated by Congress. The U.S. Government Accountability Office (GAO) issued two studies that provide an overview of limited-service hospitals. The first report analyzed market share, physician ownership, and patients served. The second covered geographic location, services provided, and financial performance.[12] The Medicare Payment Advisory Commission weighed in on the issue of specialty hospitals with a report to Congress in March 2005.[13] Finally, the Centers for Medicare & Medicaid Services (CMS) completed a mandated study of physician-owned specialty hospitals.[14]

Both GAO reports summarize the arguments for and against limited-service hospitals, which they refer to as *specialty hospitals.* Proponents contend that specialty hospitals provide more efficient delivery of high-quality specialty services, and individual patients generally experience greater comfort and convenience. Physicians enjoy financial and work environment advantages, more

control over patient scheduling and equipment purchasing, and greater financial gains through increased productivity and ownership interests. Critics argue that specialty hospitals are skimming off the more financially rewarding service lines and patients from general hospitals, that patients admitted to specialty hospitals are less critically ill than those seen in a general hospital, and that physician ownership of these specialty hospitals may inappropriately influence physicians' clinical and referral behavior. The reports also discuss the smaller number of Medicaid patients treated at specialty hospitals and the absence of emergency departments in more than half of them.

Congress responded to the concerns about limited-service providers by authorizing a moratorium that blocked physicians from referring patients to certain types of specialty hospitals in which they have an ownership or investment interest. The 18-month moratorium expired in June 2005, but it has been extended by a de facto regulatory ban by the Centers for Medicare & Medicaid Services. This ban is intended to remain in place until CMS completes a review of Medicare payment policies.[15]

Teaching Hospitals

What is a teaching hospital?

A teaching hospital offers residency training to physicians through affiliation with a medical school. Teaching hospitals may also have accredited programs for training nurses or allied health personnel. There are nearly 1,500 teaching hospitals in the United States, of which about 400 are considered to be major teaching hospitals by the Association of American Medical College's Council on Teaching Hospitals.[16]

How many medical schools and academic medical centers are there?

There are 125 accredited medical schools that grant the MD degree, according to the Association of American Medical Colleges. Additionally, there are 20 schools that grant the DO (Doctor of Osteopathy) degree, according to the American Association of Colleges of Osteopathic Medicine.[17] Academic medical centers consist of a university hospital and medical school. They may also include associated hospitals and clinics, other professional training programs, research organizations and laboratories, and libraries, thereby linking research, medical education training, and patient care.[18]

Table 3–2.	Beds and Utilization: U.S. Registered Community Hospitals, 1975–2004		
Year	Hospitals	Beds	Admissions
1975	5,875	942,000	33,435,000
1980	5,830	988,000	36,143,000
1990	5,384	927,000	31,181,000
2000	4,915	824,000	33,089,000
2004	4,919	808,000	35,086,000

Source: AHA Hospital Statistics, 2006 ed. (Chicago: Health Forum, 2006): 4.

Table 3–4.	Outpatient Visits to U.S. Registered Community Hospitals, 1975–2004
Year	Outpatient Visits
1975	190,672,000
1980	202,310,000
1990	301,329,000
2000	521,404,000
2004	571,569,000

Source: AHA Hospital Statistics, 2006 ed. (Chicago: Health Forum, 2006): 4.

Utilization Trends

Is inpatient utilization declining?

The total number of community hospitals and the number of community hospital beds have decreased since the mid-1970s, as shown in table 3–2. For a while, the number of inpatient admissions to community hospitals also decreased. Due to the influence of managed care, among other factors, total inpatient admissions to community hospitals dropped in the early 1990s. More recently, however, admissions have begun to increase, totaling 35 million in 2004. Another way to look at admissions data is as the ratio of *admissions per 1,000 population*. For community hospitals, this utilization metric has declined dramatically, from about 160 admissions per 1,000 in 1980 to the current rate of about 120 per 1,000, which has held relatively unchanged over the past 10 years.[19]

Is length of stay declining?

Another key inpatient utilization indicator is *average length of stay*, which measures how long a patient stays in the hospital once admitted. Over the past 30 years, the average length of stay in community hospitals has been shortened by two full days, from just under eight days in 1975 to just under six days in 2004, as shown in table 3–3.

Table 3–3.	Average Length of Stay: U.S. Registered Community Hospitals, 1975–2004
Year	Average Length of Stay (Days)
1975	7.7
1980	7.6
1990	7.2
2000	5.8
2004	5.6

Source: AHA Hospital Statistics, 2006 ed. (Chicago: Health Forum, 2006): 4.

What will happen in the future?

The factors likely to have the greatest impact on utilization in the near future, particularly the growth and aging of the population and the growth of outpatient care, appear to indicate a continuation of demand for health services. Less predictable are the effects of future changes in reimbursement or other shifts in government policy, and the potential demands for care resulting from a disease outbreak or disaster-relief situation.[20]

How much outpatient care do hospitals deliver?

Total outpatient visits in U.S. hospitals have increased steadily, reaching nearly 600 million in 2004, as shown in table 3–4. Emergency-room visits and outpatient surgical procedures have also increased.

Are hospitals losing ambulatory surgery market share?

A few decades ago, hospitals had the entire market for surgery, and most of it was inpatient. Today, hospitals face competition from freestanding outpatient surgery centers, limited-service surgical hospitals, and physicians' offices for surgical market share. According to estimates from market analyst Verispan, in 2004, hospitals had 62 percent, freestanding outpatient surgery centers had 17 percent, and physicians' offices had 21 percent of the ambulatory surgery market. Yet outpatient care of all types is critically important to the financial health of the hospital, representing an estimated 60 percent of the typical hospital's operating margin.[21]

What are the major service lines in a hospital?

Major service lines in the acute care general hospital often include cardiology, oncology, orthopedics, and women's services, among others. These service lines may be developed into a full continuum of care and become centers of excellence for the hospital. They are also likely to be the focus of competition from other local providers.[22]

How many hospital beds are available?

In 2004, there were about 956,000 beds in all registered hospitals in the United States, and about 808,000 of these beds were in community hospitals. This represents a ratio of nearly three beds per 1,000 population for community hospitals.[23]

Issues

Why is patient safety a big issue now?

Consumers are participating in their own health care in greater numbers. This includes selecting quality health care organizations that are also working to improve their quality. A hospital's reputation and accountability influence consumer decisions. Meanwhile, medical errors drive up liability insurance, for both providers and physicians, and thereby, the costs of care.

What are the national patient safety goals?

The Joint Commission on the Accreditation of Healthcare Organizations developed National Patient Safety Goals. These program-specific goals were developed for 2004, with additions each subsequent year, for all accreditation programs. The purpose is to promote specific improvements in patient safety. The goals highlight problems and present evidence- and expert-based solutions.[24]

For hospitals, through 2005, these goals included:

- Improving the accuracy of patient identification
- Improving the effectiveness of communication among caregivers
- Improving the safety of using medications
- Improving the safety of using infusion pumps
- Reducing the risk of health care-associated infections
- Accurately and completely reconciling medications across the continuum of care
- Reducing the risk of patient harm resulting from falls[25]

Is it possible to compare hospitals based on patient outcomes data?

Although other factors also influence the choice of a particular hospital, many consumers place confidence in the traditional sources of information— recommendations by their personal physicians and the experiences of family and friends. For many consumers, choice of the hospital is also governed by insurance considerations, where their physicians have privileges, and how far they are willing to travel for care.[26]

Over the past 25 years, a number of initiatives have been established to collect and report comparative data on patient outcomes at different hospitals to allow more informed choices by consumers, employers, and health plans. In the mid-1980s, the Health Care Financing Administration (HCFA), the former name of the federal agency responsible for administering the Medicare and Medicaid programs, began to collect comparative hospital mortality data. Although it was later discontinued, this initiative was followed by other data-collection and reporting projects intended to allow the comparison of hospitals based on performance indicators such as death rates or complication rates. Among the most well-known of these later initiatives are the *U.S. News & World Report* listing of best hospitals and the Solucient *100 Top Hospitals*.[27] Another key initiative is the *Hospital Compare* database on the Centers for Medicare & Medicaid Services website. This interactive website allows consumers to evaluate some 4,000 hospitals based on measures related to heart attack, heart failure, and pneumonia patients, as well as on surgical infection prevention.[28]

How are rural hospitals doing?

Some experts believe that rural hospitals need their own rural-specific quality indicators to measure the unique and common aspects of services they provide. They argue that current measurements by the government and private sector cannot accurately or fairly quantify the level of care provided at rural facilities.[29]

Why are some hospitals tax exempt?

Under current law, hospitals may be exempt from taxes because of their community benefit; they promote the health of residents in their community. Tax exemption is considered a subsidy for the costs federal and local governments would incur by providing health services. Charity care is not the only justification of hospitals' tax-exempt status, according to IRS Revenue Ruling 69-545 (1969). The promotion of health care is itself a charitable activity.[30]

Ambulatory Care Centers

As more health care services have moved out of the traditional hospital setting, the variety and number of ambulatory care facilities has grown.

Among the most common services now offered in freestanding facilities are ambulatory surgery and diagnostic imaging.

Ambulatory Surgery Centers

What are the origins of ambulatory surgery?

The first ambulatory surgery centers (ASCs) opened in 1969. Growth was slow until 1982, when Medicare approved reimbursement for ambulatory surgery centers. This triggered substantial growth. Health plans also encouraged the growth of ASCs, which they found attractive because of the lower costs of care in the outpatient surgery center setting. Today, nearly 70 percent of all surgeries are done on an outpatient basis.[31]

How many ambulatory surgery centers are there, and who owns them?

As of 2002, there were more than 3,500 Medicare-certified ambulatory surgery centers in the United States. Ambulatory Surgery Centers can be owned by hospitals, physicians, or management companies. For hospitals, offering ambulatory surgery frees up surgical space for larger-scale surgical programs, generates profits, and provides a site for higher-quality outpatient surgical services. It also provides options for joint ventures with physicians. For physicians, ASCs provide practice convenience, operating site control, and profit.

Diagnostic Imaging Centers

What types of technology do you find in diagnostic imaging centers?

Technology has been the driving force behind the increase in outpatient diagnostic imaging services. Diagnostic imaging centers offer a variety of services, including magnetic resonance imaging (MRI), computed tomography (CT), nuclear medicine, ultrasound, mammography, radiography and fluoroscopy, MR angiography, bone densitometry, and cardiac stress testing.[32]

Who owns diagnostic imaging centers, and how many are there?

Diagnostic imaging centers are owned by hospitals, physicians, cardiologists, obstetricians, radiologists, and for-profit companies.[33] In 2000, there were slightly more than 3,300 diagnostic imaging centers.[34]

Urgent-Care Centers

What role do urgent-care centers plan?

The first urgent-care centers opened about 20 years ago, and the industry has seen rapid growth.[35] Urgent-care centers are ambulatory care centers that are usually open 7 days a week for 13 to 24 hours. Urgent-care centers serve walk-in patients; that is, they do not require an appointment. They offer an array of services including x-rays, laboratory testing, on-site pharmacy, procedure rooms for lacerations and fracture care, exam rooms, and specialized corporate services for employee health and workers' compensation cases.

Because many injuries and illnesses are acute and non–life-threatening, and happen to otherwise healthy people, these patients can seek services at urgent-care centers rather than at emergency departments. This keeps costs down while allowing emergency department staff to attend to true emergencies. Also, injuries or illnesses do not always occur during regular physician office hours. Urgent-care centers fill the gap.[36]

Long-Term Care Facilities

Long-term care covers a broad range of services of varying complexity and intensity, but the term generally refers to care that will take place over a month or longer—in many cases, much longer. At one end of the continuum are supportive services, such as home-maker or adult day care, intended to help people remain in their own homes. At the more intensive end of the continuum is care in a nursing facility or long-term hospital. Some long-term care services are provided to patients who will eventually return to full health and independence, but many are provided to frail or chronically ill elderly patients who will need care for the rest of their lives. With the aging of the American population, the demand for long-term care services of all types is likely to increase.

Nursing Homes

What types of nursing homes are there?

The term *nursing home* recalls the early days of the industry, when mansions or other large houses were converted into facilities for the elderly. The Social Security Act of 1965, which created the Medicare and Medicaid programs, introduced two levels of nursing home care: skilled nursing and intermediate care. As originally set up, skilled nursing facilities were eligible for reimbursement under both programs, but intermediate-care facilities (ICFs) could only participate in Medicaid. Although at the federal level the term *intermediate-care facility* was later changed to *nursing facility*, the ICF category is retained by some state licensure laws.

Table 3–5. Number of Nursing Facilities and Beds, 2000–2005

	2000	2001	2002	2003	2004	2005
Beds	1,702,973	1,702,622	1,696,201	1,694,889	1,683,068	1,678,306
Facilities	16,765	16,652	16,486	16,347	16,121	16,032

Source: U.S. Centers for Medicare & Medicaid Services, OSCAR data, cited in American Health Care Association, *Trends in Certified Nursing Facilities, Beds and Patients* (2005), http://www.ahca.org/research/oscar/trend_graph_facilities_beds_patients_200506.pdf (accessed June 30, 2005).

Skilled nursing care is the more intensive type of nursing home care, and it can be provided in a freestanding facility or as a distinct part of another institution, such as a hospital. Under Medicare regulations, a skilled nursing facility is required to have a transfer agreement in effect with at least one hospital and provide either skilled nursing care or rehabilitation services. Another key Medicare requirement for skilled nursing facilities is supervision by a registered nurse and the provision of licensed nursing care on a 24-hour basis. Intermediate-care facilities provide a less intensive level of care.[37]

How many nursing homes are there?

As of 2005, there were about 16,000 nursing facilities certified for participation in the Medicare and Medicaid programs—about 700 fewer than five years earlier. The number of beds in these nursing facilities has held fairly steady at about 1.7 million over this five-year period, as shown in table 3–5. Approximately two-thirds of certified nursing facilities are for-profit, and some are part of nursing facility chains. The largest nursing home operators in 2004 were Manor Care, Beverly Enterprises, and Kindred Healthcare, all for-profit and publicly traded.[38]

Other Types of Long-Term Care

What are assisted living and other alternatives to nursing home care?

Assisted living facilities are for people who need assistance with the routine activities of daily living, such as bathing, dressing, and eating. They encourage independence and provide less intensive care than traditional nursing facilities.[39] Alternatives to nursing home care, besides assisted living, include continuing-care retirement communities, adult day care centers, and home health care.[40]

What is the hospital's role in long-term care and senior housing?

Some hospitals offer a nursing-home–type unit or facility. These can include skilled nursing, intermediate care, personal care, and sheltered or residential care.[41]

Health Systems and Networks

Many hospitals are part of a larger group through ownership, contract management, or affiliation agreements. These larger groups may be multi-institutional systems, such as Catholic Health Initiatives (with 56 hospitals), or networks, like the Central Virginia Health Network (with nine members).[42] Since the first attempts to identify and survey them in the early 1970s, the number of health systems and their hospitals has increased.

Health Systems

What is a health system?

According to the American Hospital Association, both multi-hospital systems and single hospital systems exist: "A multihospital health care system is two or more hospitals owned, leased, sponsored, or contract managed by a central organization," whereas "single, freestanding member hospitals may be categorized a health care systems by bringing into membership three or more, and at least 25 percent, of their owned or leased non-hospital preacute and postacute health care organizations."[43]

How did the trend toward system building begin?

For many years, hospitals could be categorized as a cottage industry in which individual providers were largely independent of each other. The trend toward system building began in the 1960s with the rise of investor-owned companies that acquired existing hospitals or built new ones. The cost-based Medicare reimbursement system in place at the time helped these companies achieve success in many markets. Not-for-profit hospital system growth began in earnest in the mid-1970s, partly in reaction to competition from the for-profit chains and partly due to a changing regulatory environment, among other factors.[44]

What are the organizational models for systems?

The AHA's Health Research and Education Trust, along with the University of California–Berkeley, developed an identification system for systems. There are five categories based on the degree of differentiation or centralization of hospital services, physician arrangements, and provider-based insurance products. *Centralization* refers to the amount of decision making and service delivery that emanates from the system level instead of from the individual hospitals.

These categories are:

- Centralized health system
- Centralized physician/insurance health system
- Moderately centralized health system
- Decentralized health system
- Independent hospital system[45]

How many systems are there, and how many hospitals and beds are in systems?

Based on AHA membership data, there are 357 multi-hospital health care systems in the United States.[46] These systems are composed of 3,297 hospitals and 586,594 beds.[47]

Networks

What is a network, and how many are there?

The American Hospital Association defines networks as "a group of hospitals, physicians, other providers, insurers and/or community agencies that work together to coordinate and deliver a broad spectrum of services to their community."[48] There are 152 networks in the United States today.

Mergers and Acquisitions

Is it a merger, an acquisition, or an affiliation?

A merger is the combination of two or more entities into a single entity so that only one of the companies survives as a legal entity. In an acquisition, one entity comes into possession or control of another entity. An affiliation brings together two or more entities as members, associates, or branches to coordinate and integrate activities without completely merging or consolidating.

What have the trends been with hospital mergers and acquisitions?

In the 1990s, there was a dramatic increase in the number of mergers and acquisitions of hospitals. Many of these agreements were the result of financial concerns and consolidation of services. Since 1998, however, this trend has slowed as mergers have dropped from a high of 310 in 1997 to a steady 86 in 2000, 83 in 2001, 58 in 2002, 38 in 2003, and then a slight increase to 55 in 2004. Hospital mergers and acquisitions are projected to remain sluggish.[49]

References

1. Albert V. Whitehall and Bremen I. Johnson, "Putting S. 191 to Work," *Hospitals* 20, no. 9 (September 1946): 35–38.
2. Caroline Rossi Steinberg, "Trends: An Overview of 2004," in American Hospital Association, *AHA Hospital Statistics*, 2006 ed. (Chicago: Health Forum, 2006): viii–xiv.
3. Ellen Heath Grinney, *The Hospital* (New York: Chelsea House, 1991): 13–38.
4. *AHA Hospital Statistics*: 6.
5. U.S. Department of Justice and U.S. Federal Trade Commission, "Industry Snapshot: Hospitals," in *Improving Health Care: A Dose of Competition* (July 2004): 3, http://www.usdoj.gov/atr/public/health_care/204694.pdf (accessed June 27, 2005); American College of Surgeons Committee on Trauma, *Resources for Optimal Care of the Injured Patient: 1999* (Chicago, American College of Surgeons, 1998): 99–102; American Academy of Pediatrics Committee on Fetus and Newborn, "Levels of Neonatal Care," *Pediatrics* 114, no. 5 (November 2004): 1341–1347, http://pediatrics.aappublications.org/cgi/content/full/114/5/1341 (accessed November 15, 2005).
6. Alan M. Zuckerman, "Creating Competitive Advantage: Product Development," *Healthcare Financial Management* 59, no. 6 (June 2005): 110, 112, 114; Kristen Hallam, "Doctors Fear Excellence Designation," *Modern Healthcare* (December 18, 2000): 30; U.S. Centers for Medicare & Medicaid Services, *Medicare Partnerships for Quality Services Demonstration* (2004), http://www.cms.hhs.gov/researchers/demos/mpqsdem.asp (accessed June 27, 2005); U.S. Department of Health and Human Services, Office on Women's Health, *National Centers of Excellence in Women's Health*, http://www.4woman.gov/COE/index.htm (accessed June 27, 2005).
7. U.S. Centers for Medicare & Medicaid Services, *Critical Access Hospital Program: Fact Sheet* (December 2004), http://www.cms.hhs.gov/medlearn/2CritAccssHospProfctsht.pdf (accessed June 28, 2005); American Hospital Association, *CAH Update* (May 2005), http://www.aha.org/aha/key_issues/rural/content/2005mayupdatecah.pdf (accessed November 10, 2005); American Hospital Association, "Critical Access Hospital Growth," (January 2005), http://www.aha.org/aha/key_issues/rural/content/050124cahgrowth.pdf (accessed June 28, 2005).

8. National Association of Public Hospitals and Health Systems, *NAPH Issue Brief: What is a Safety Net Hospital?* (Washington, DC: NAPH, 2004), http://www.naph.org/Content/NavigationMenu/About_Our_Members/Frequently_Asked_Questions1/IB_2004_9_What_is.pdf (accessed June 28, 2005).

9. Charles N. Kahn, "Intolerable Risk, Irreparable Harm: The Legacy of Physician-Owned Specialty Hospitals," *Health Affairs* 25, no. 1 (January–February 2006): 130–133.

10. American Hospital Association, "Impact of Limited-Service Providers on Communities and Full-Service Hospitals," *Trend Watch* 6, no. 2 (September 2004): 1, http://www.ahapolicyforum.org/ahapolicyforum/trendwatch/content/040924_twvol6no2limitedserv.pdf (accessed June 28, 2005).

11. Missouri Hospital Association, "Limited Service Providers: An Overview," *Briefing Paper* 1 (January 2005), http://web.mhanet.com/asp/governmental_relations/pdf/lsp/overview.pdf (accessed June 28, 2005); Stuart Guterman, "Specialty Hospitals: A Problem or a Symptom?" *Health Affairs* 25, no. 1 (January–February 2006): 95–105.

12. A. Bruce Steinwald et al., *Specialty Hospitals: Information on National Market Share, Physician Ownership, and Patients Served* (Washington, DC: U.S. General Accounting Office, April 18, 2003), http://www.gao.gov/new.items/d03683r.pdf (accessed May 14, 2005); A. Bruce Steinwald et al., *Specialty Hospitals: Geographic Location, Services Provided, and Financial Performance.* (Washington, DC: U.S. GAO, October 2003), http://www.gao.gov/new.items/d04167.pdf (accessed May 14, 2005).

13. Medicare Payment Advisory Commission. *Report to the Congress: Physician-Owned Specialty Hospitals* (Washington, DC: MedPAC, March 2005), http://www.medpac.gov/publications/congressional_reports/Mar05_SpecHospitals.pdf?CFID=1360124&CFTOKEN=54936215 (accessed May 14, 2005).

14. U.S. Centers for Medicare & Medicaid Services, *Study of Physician-Owned Specialty Hospitals Required in Section 507(c)(2) of the Medicare Prescription Drug, Improvement, and Modernization Act of 2003* (2005), http://www.cms.hhs.gov/media/press/files/052005/RTC-StudyofPhysOwnedSpecHosp.pdf (accessed September 29, 2005).

15. Chris Serb, "Moratorium Redux," *Hospitals & Health Networks* 79, no. 10 (October 2005): 12, http://www.hhnmag.com/hhnmag/hospitalconnect/search/article.jsp?dcrpath=HHNMAG/PubsNewsArticle/data/0510HHN_Inbox_Legislation&domain=HHNMAG (accessed November 7, 2005).

16. American Hospital Association, *Annual Survey Database: For Fiscal Year 2004 Data* (Chicago: Health Forum, 2006).

17. American Association of Medical Colleges, *Teaching Hospitals*, http://www.aamc.org/medicalschools.htm (accessed June 28, 2005); American Association of Colleges of Osteopathic Medicine, Office of Research and Information Services, telephone conversation, June 28, 2005.

18. Joint Commission on Accreditation of Healthcare Organizations, *Lexikon*, 2nd ed. (Oakbrook Terrace, IL: Joint Commission on Accreditation of Healthcare Organizations, 1998): 1.

19. *AHA Hospital Statistics*: viii.

20. American Hospital Association, The Lewin Group, "Forces Driving Inpatient Utilization," *TrendWatch* 3, no. 3 (November 2001): 2, http://www.ahapolicyforum.org/ahapolicyforum/trendwatch/content/twnov2001.pdf (accessed June 28, 2005); William J. Scanlon, "The Future of Medicare Hospital Payment," *Health Affairs* 25, no. 1 (January–February 2006): 70–80.

21. Yasmine Iqbal, "Can Hospitals Keep Their Share of the Outpatient Surgery Market?" *Outpatient Surgery Magazine* 5, no. 6 (June 2004), http://www.outpatientsurgery.net/2004/os06/hospitals_keep_share_outpatient_market.php (accessed June 28, 2005).

22. Alan M. Zuckerman and Tracy K. Johnson, "Filling Gaps in the Continuum," *Health Progress* 82, no. 6 (November–December 2001): 34–38.

23. *AHA Hospital Statistics*: 2, 4, 11.

24. Joint Commission on Accreditation of Healthcare Organizations, *National Patient Safety Goals for 2005 and 2004*, http://www.jcaho.org/accredited+organizations/patient+safety/npsg.htm (accessed June 28, 2005).

25. Joint Commission on Accreditation of Healthcare Organizations, *2005 Hospitals' National Patient Safety Goals*, http://www.jcaho.org/accredited+organizations/patient+safety/05+npsg/05_npsg_hap.htm (accessed June 28, 2005).

26. Ian Morrison, "Quality Information: Are Consumers Ready for Report Cards?" *Hospitals & Health Networks* 77, no. 4 (April 2003): 38, 40, http://www.hhnmag.com/hhnmag/hospitalconnect/search/article.jsp?dcrpath=AHA/PubsNewsArticle/data/0304HHN_CoverStory_SB_Quality&domain=HHNMAG (accessed November 9, 2005).

27. Solucient, *100 Top Hospitals*, http://www.100tophospitals.com (accessed November 9, 2005); "Best Hospitals 2005," *U.S. News & World Report* (July 18, 2005), http://www.usnews.com/usnews/health/best-hospitals/tophosp.htm (accessed November 9, 2005).

28. U.S. Centers for Medicare & Medicaid Services, *Hospital Compare.* http://www.hospitalcompare.hhs.gov (accessed November 9, 2005).

29. Joseph Mantone, "Special Report: Rural Route," *Modern Healthcare* 35, no. 20 (May 16, 2005): 28–29, 34; Ira Moscovice et al., "Measuring Rural Hospital Quality," *The Journal of Rural Health* 20, no. 4 (Fall 2004): 383–393.

30. Healthcare Financial Management Association, *HFMA Wants You to Know: P&P Board Examines the Relationship of Community Benefit to Hospital Tax-Exempt Status* (April 20, 2005), http://www.hfma.org/publications/ HFMA_WantsYouToKnow/042005.htm (accessed June 28, 2005).

31. Scott Becker et al., *Ambulatory Surgery Centers: Legal and Regulatory Issues,* 2nd ed. (Washington, DC: America Health Lawyers Association, 2003): 1–2.

32. *The Directory of Independent Ambulatory Care Centers,* 2002 ed. (Millerton, NY: Grey House Publishing, 2002).

33. Thomas E. Bartrum, *Diagnostic Imaging Centers: Legal and Regulatory Issues* (Washington, DC: American Health Lawyers Association, 2003): 10.

34. Ibid: 9.

35. Urgent Care Association of America, *Urgent Care,* http://www.ucaoa.org/urgent_care.htm (accessed June 28, 2005).

36. North American Association for Ambulatory Urgent Care, *Frequently Asked Questions,* http://www.nafac.com/ faqs.php (accessed June 20, 2005).

37. U.S. Centers for Medicare & Medicaid Services, "Requirements for States and Long Term Care Facilities," *Code of Federal Regulations* title 42, part 483 (October 1, 2004), http://www.access.gpo.gov/ nara/cfr/waisidx_04/42cfr483_04.html (accessed June 30, 2005); Mark A. Hall, ed., *Health Care Corporate Law: Facilities and Transactions* (Boston: Little, Brown and Co., 1996): 7-8–7-9.

38. American Association of Homes and Services for the Aging, *Aging Services: The Facts,* http://www.aahsa.org/ aging_services/default.asp (accessed November 9, 2005); U.S. Centers for Medicare & Medicaid Services, OSCAR data, cited in American Health Care Association, *Trends in Certified Nursing Facilities, Beds and Patients* (2005), http://www.ahca.org/ research/oscar/trend_graph_facilities_ beds_patients_200506.pdf (accessed June 30, 2005); Kathleen Vickery, "Top 50 Nursing Facility Chains & Top 40 Assisted Living Chains, 2004," *Provider* 31, no. 6 (June 2005): 45–49.

39. Joint Commission on Accreditation of Healthcare Organizations, *Lexikon*: 18.

40. American Association of Homes and Services for the Aging, *Aging Services.*

41. *AHA Hospital Statistics*: 199.

42. American Hospital Association, *AHA Guide to the Health Care Field,* 2006 ed. (Chicago: Health Forum, 2006): B25, B153.

43. *AHA Guide to the Health Care Field,* 2006 ed. (Chicago: Health Forum, 2006): B2.

44. Stephen M. Shortell, "The Evolution of Hospital Systems: Unfulfilled Promises and Self-fulfilling Prophesies," *Medical Care Review* 45, no. 2 (Fall 1988): 177–214; Alison Evans Cuellar and Paul J. Gertler, "Trends in Hospital Consolidation: The Formation of Local Systems," *Health Affairs* 22, no. 6 (November–December 2003): 77–87.

45. *AHA Guide to the Health Care Field*: B2.

46. Ibid.: B3.

47. Ibid.: B3.

48. Ibid.: B2.

49. Modern Healthcare, *By the Numbers* (December 20, 2004): 6, http://www.modernhealthcare.com/ docs/bythenumbers04.pdf (accessed June 24, 2005).

No longer will older Americans be denied the healing miracle of modern medicine. No longer will illness crush and destroy the savings that they have so carefully put away over a lifetime so that they might enjoy dignity in their later years.

(Lyndon B. Johnson, July 1965, on signing the Medicare legislation)

Health care in the United States is financed through private health insurance, primarily employer-sponsored, and public entitlement programs, most notably Medicare and Medicaid. This country is unique among developed nations in its reliance on the private sector for both funding and delivering health care. However, Medicare and Medicaid programs have grown so much since their inception in the 1960s that the federal government is now the largest payor for hospital care.

Most developed countries offer some form of universal health care, but the models for financing and delivering health care vary. The United Kingdom, for example, provides universal health care directly through its tax-supported National Health Service. The Canadian model also offers tax-supported universal health care, but provides care indirectly through private providers that are reimbursed through its single-payor system. The German health system is based on a compulsory insurance model for universal care. Private insurance remains available in all three countries to supplement public financing. Regardless of the national model, all health systems are challenged to balance access and quality issues with costs.[1]

This chapter will cover trends in national health spending and the costs of health care. The roles of both the public and private payors (Medicare, Medicaid, and private insurers), and what they mean for hospitals, will also be examined.

Health Spending

How much do we spend as a nation on health care?

The nation spent nearly $1.7 trillion on health care in 2003. National health expenditures may rise to over $1.9 trillion in 2005 and $3.5 trillion by 2014. In other words, over $5,600 was spent per person in 2003. By 2014 the per-capita expenditure is projected to be $11,000.[2]

How much of the gross domestic product does this represent?

National health expenditures represented 15 percent of the gross domestic product (GDP) in 2003. Experts expect this percentage to climb to nearly 19 percent by 2014. U.S. spending on health care, as a percentage of GDP, exceeds that of any other country. According to the international Organisation for Economic Co-operation and Development, which represents the world's major developed countries, health expenditures in member countries averaged 8.6 percent of GDP in 2003. Although the United States tops the world in health care spending, developed countries that spend less may have comparable or better health status, as indicated by measures such as infant mortality and life expectancy. However, health care costs have been rising at comparable rates in all developed countries.[3]

How is the nation's health dollar allocated among sectors?

In 2003 hospital care claimed the largest share of national health expenditures, with 31 percent of the total, as shown in figure 4–1. Physician and clinical services accounted for 22 percent, nursing home care for 7 percent, and prescription drugs for 11 percent. The private sector paid for 55 percent of national health expenditures, while the other 45 percent came from Medicare, Medicaid, and other public sources.[4]

WHERE IT CAME FROM

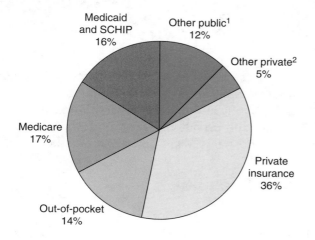

WHERE IT WENT

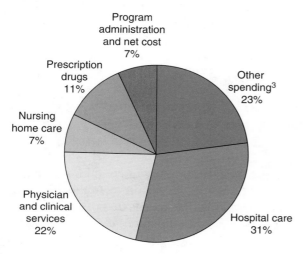

Figure 4–1. The nation's health dollar, 2003.

Source: Centers for Medicare & Medicaid Services, Office of the Actuary, National Health Statistics Group, *The Nation's Health Dollar: 2003* (January 11, 2005), http://www.cms.hhs.gov/statistics/nhe/historical/chart.asp (accessed February 25, 2005).

What are the trends in out-of-pocket spending by consumers?

Consumer out-of-pocket payments accounted for 14 percent of all national health spending in 2003. This amounted to just under $500 for each person, an increase of about 8 percent from 2002. For the typical senior citizen, out-of-pocket health care spending has been estimated at roughly $3,500 per year.[5]

What do spending projections reveal?

Growth in health care spending has been outpacing the economy. From 2002 to 2003 health expenditures grew by just under 8 percent, a slower rate than the 9 percent growth of the previous 12 months, but greater than the 5 percent annual

growth in the nation's GDP for 2003. Health expenditures have been shifting proportionally from the private to the public sector, with government's share expected to amount to nearly half of all health spending by 2014.[6]

Why are health care costs rising?

Rising health care costs can be attributed to many factors, whose relative importance varies with the perspective of the industry sector. To health insurers, for instance, the culprit is hospital costs. But what's causing hospital costs to increase? Key cost drivers for the health industry at large include the following:

- Inflation
- Population growth and aging
- Increased case complexity and intensity of services (number and kinds of services used)
- Advances in medical technology
- Higher labor costs due to increasing specialization of the labor force and a shortage of nurses and other health care workers[7]

Key cost drivers for hospitals are shown in figure 4–2.

Financing Health Care

Overview

The U.S. health care system traditionally has been based on voluntary, private health insurance, with multiple payors and sources of coverage. Many Americans are insured by employer-based group health plans, but there are a significant number of uninsured and underinsured individuals as well as disparities in access and coverage. The public insurance programs, Medicare and Medicaid, have grown in importance since their introduction 40 years ago. Addressing rising costs remain a challenge for both the private and public sectors.

The complexity of the U.S. health system adds to its administrative costs and makes reform difficult, but the system's diversity spurs technological advancement and allows for consumer choice.[8]

Medicare

What are the origins of Medicare?

Medicare was enacted in 1965 as part of the Social Security Act, creating an entitlement program to provide health coverage to most Americans over the age of 65. By the end of the first year, 19 million had enrolled. Several years later, services were extended to younger individuals with long-term

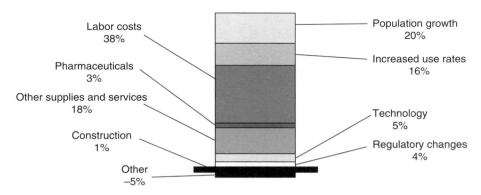

Figure 4–2. Share of growth in spending on hospital care, 2001–2003 projected.

Source: PricewaterhouseCoopers, *Cost of Caring: Key Drivers of Growth in Spending on Hospital Care* (American Hospital Association and the Federation of American Hospitals, February 19, 2003), http://www.aha.org/aha/press_room-info/content/PwCcostsReport.pdf (accessed June 27, 2005).

disabilities or end-stage renal disease. While other modifications in the Medicare program have been made, the most significant expansion came with the Medicare Prescription Drug, Improvement, and Modernization Act (MMA), which became law in 2003. MMA added the new outpatient prescription drug benefit, effective in 2006.[9]

How is Medicare structured and funded?

The four parts of the Medicare program, and their funding sources, are as follows:

- Part A, the Hospital Insurance (HI) program, covers inpatient hospital, outpatient diagnostic services, and post-hospitalization skilled nursing facility, hospice, and home health care. Employees and employers each pay a 1.45 percent payroll tax to finance this program.
- Part B, Supplementary Medical Insurance (SMI), covers physician and outpatient therapeutic care, lab tests, medical supplies, and home health. It's financed by beneficiary premiums (25 percent) and general federal tax revenues (75 percent).
- Part C, Medicare Advantage, refers to private managed care plans that provide Part A and B benefits to enrollees. Funding for Part C is the same as that for Parts A and B.
- Part D relates to the outpatient prescription drug benefit. Funding will be through general federal tax revenues, premiums charged beneficiaries, and state payments.[10]

The Medicare program is administered by the Centers for Medicare & Medicaid Services

(CMS), part of the U.S. Department of Health and Human Services.

How many are covered by Medicare, and who is eligible?

Medicare currently covers over 41 million Americans. Coverage is available to senior citizens primarily. However, younger people with disabilities are also eligible and comprise 14 percent of Medicare beneficiaries.[11]

Medicare Part A hospital insurance coverage is available free for people over age 65 or the disabled who qualify for Social Security benefits. Senior citizens not meeting Social Security eligibility requirements may enroll by paying a Part A premium of up to $375 per month in 2005. For all beneficiaries, an annual deductible of $912 applies for a 2005 hospital stay of 60 days or less. Costly co-payments apply for extended hospital or skilled nursing facility stays.[12]

All participants pay for Part B Medicare coverage. The monthly Part B premium in 2005 was $78.20. There was also a $110 annual deductible in 2005 and a 20 percent beneficiary co-payment for most Part B services.[13]

Part C Medicare Advantage managed-care plan participation is available in many parts of the country. Enrollees of both Part A and B coverage may opt to participate in a Medicare Advantage private health plan to receive their Medicare-covered benefits. These plans may offer additional benefits and other choices, and there may be an extra monthly premium for the enhanced benefits.[14]

For Part D prescription drug benefits, coverage is to be provided by private companies that have contracted with Medicare. A variety of plans with different costs will be available to Medicare enrollees on a voluntary basis.[15]

What is supplemental Medicare coverage?

Medicare does not cover all medical services, and Medicare deductibles and other cost sharing can become costly. According to the Kaiser Family Foundation, Medicare covered less than half (45 percent) of beneficiaries' health care costs in 2002. Seniors may rely on employer-sponsored retiree health benefits, privately purchased Medigap insurance, Medicare Advantage plans, or Medicaid to cover the "gaps" in their Medicare coverage.[16]

The availability of employer-sponsored retiree health benefits has been eroding in recent years. The number of large employers offering retiree benefits declined from 66 percent to 36 percent between 1988 and 2004, and this trend is expected to continue.[17]

Medigap insurance is sold by private insurance companies, but a policy offered must conform, in most cases, to one of the ten standardized sets of benefits mandated by federal law. Labeled A to J, these Medigap policies offer a range from basic to more comprehensive benefits.[18]

Medicare Part C's Medicare Advantage managed-care plans may offer enrollees additional benefits for an added cost.

Medicare participants with very low incomes may also qualify for Medicaid assistance in paying for Medicare premiums, deductibles, and co-payments, and for services not covered by Medicare. These individuals are often referred to as dual eligibles.

More than 90 percent of Medicare beneficiaries relied on supplemental coverage in 2001. Retiree health benefits accounted for 31 percent of this coverage, Medigap policies for 26 percent, Medicare Advantage plans for 16 percent, and Medicaid for 15 percent.[19]

How is Medicare spending allocated?

In 2005 Medicare is expected to spend $325 billion in benefits. Part A benefits account for 45 percent of Medicare expenditures, Part B for 35 percent, and Part C for 15 percent. Administrative costs for Medicare have been estimated at less than 2 percent each for Part A and Part B programs.[20]

What is the prospective payment system?

In an effort to control costs and promote efficiency, the federal government introduced the inpatient acute hospital prospective payment system (PPS) in 1983. With the inpatient PPS, hospitals are paid for treatment of Medicare patients based on predetermined flat rates instead of being reimbursed for costs.

Some facilities were originally excluded from the prospective payment system. These included rehabilitation, psychiatric, long-term care, pediatric, and cancer hospitals. These hospitals continued to be paid under an amendment to Social Security law called the Tax Equity and Fiscal Responsibility Act (TEFRA) and thus became known as TEFRA facilities.[21] However, separate PPSs to cover inpatient and outpatient rehabilitation, inpatient psychiatric, and long-term hospital care, as well as skilled nursing facility services, home health services, and hospital outpatient care, have recently been implemented or are in development.

Other types of hospitals may be paid on a cost-based reimbursement basis rather than the prospective payment system. These include limited-service hospitals in rural areas, known as critical-access hospitals (see chapter 3).[22]

What are DRGs, APCs, and HIPPS codes?

To implement the prospective payment system for inpatient acute hospital care, categories known as diagnosis-related groups (DRGs) were developed for setting reimbursement rates to hospitals for the care provided to Medicare patients. There are currently over 500 DRGs used to classify medical conditions, and these are reviewed and adjusted annually.

Each inpatient is assigned a DRG, based on diagnosis, age, gender, and complications. PPS reimbursement rates are based on the average cost for treating a patient in a given DRG. The DRG base payment rate has labor and non-labor components. The labor share is adjusted using a wage index based on the geographic location of the hospital. Add-on payments are made to the base DRG rate in each of the following situations:

- The hospital treats a large percentage of low-income patients. This is the disproportionate share hospital (DSH) add-on.
- The case's cost is unusually high. Known as an outlier case, it may be eligible for additional payment.
- The hospital is an approved teaching facility. This add-on is called the indirect medical education (IME) adjustment.

In addition to the IME adjustment to a DRG payment rate, teaching hospitals are paid for direct graduate medical education (DGME), calculated per resident. Both hospital bad debt (from nonpayment of deductibles and coinsurance) and organ procurement costs for heart, liver, lung, and kidney transplants by approved facilities continue to be reimbursed on a separate, reasonable-cost basis.[23]

With the implementation of an outpatient PPS (OPPS) in 2000, ambulatory payment classifications (APCs) were introduced for reimbursement rate setting. Health insurance prospective payments system (HIPPS) codes were yet another coding system created for reimbursing types of care delivered in skilled nursing facilities, home health agencies, and inpatient rehabilitation hospitals.[24]

How are physicians reimbursed by Medicare?

A Medicare physician fee schedule was introduced in 1992 that replaced charge-based reimbursement with a payment system incorporating a resource-based relative value scale (RBRVS). Three components are factored into the fee schedule for each medical service provided: physician work, practice expense, and malpractice insurance. Further adjustments are made for geographic differences in costs. Physician work, including the time, level of skill, and effort to provide the care involved, currently accounts for 52 percent of the RBRVS, while the practice expense component averages 44 percent. All physicians in the same geographic area receive the same payment for the same service, regardless of medical specialty. Physician fee schedules are updated annually by the CMS.[25]

What are pay-for-performance programs?

Pay-for-performance programs—often referred to as P4P—have been gaining prominence as a means for improving quality and cost-efficiency. With the passage of the MMA in 2003, hospitals must report certain quality data to the Centers for Medicare & Medicaid Services in order to qualify for the full DRG annual update payments from Medicare. Hospitals that do not submit the required data will have their payment updates reduced. Other Medicare P4P initiatives are being developed and tested. Private insurers have been implementing pay-for-performance programs as well.[26]

Medicaid

What is Medicaid?

Medicaid is the major public health insurance program for low-income Americans. It was established in 1965 as a program jointly funded by federal and state governments. While the federal government establishes broad national guidelines, each state administers its own program, determining eligibility standards, the scope of services provided, and payment rates. Consequently, Medicaid coverage and reimbursement rates differ considerably from state to state.[27]

Who is eligible?

Federal law defines broad "categorically needy" groups that are eligible for Medicaid, and states have considerable latitude in determining eligibility within these groups. Generally, these groups include children, parents of dependent children, pregnant women, people with disabilities, and the elderly. All individuals within these groups must meet low-income and other guidelines, as determined by each state within federal regulations. Individual states may also expand Medicaid coverage to other "categorically related" or "medically needy" groups.

How many recipients are there?

Medicaid provided coverage in 2003 to 25 million children, 14 million adults (primarily low-income working parents), 5 million seniors, and 8 million people with disabilities—a total of over 52 million people. Low-income children and their parents comprise 75 percent of Medicaid enrollees, while the elderly and disabled represent the remaining 25 percent.

Medicaid plays a significant role in providing health care to those who would otherwise be uninsured. About one-quarter of all children rely on Medicaid for coverage, according to the Kaiser Commission on Medicaid and the Uninsured. Low-wage working families, without access to health insurance or unable to afford it, account for two-thirds of all Medicaid enrollees. Medicaid finances care for almost 60 percent of nursing home residents.

How is Medicaid funded?

Medicaid is jointly funded by the federal and state governments. The federal government share, known as the Federal Medical Assistance Percentage (FMAP), is calculated annually by means of a formula that compares each state's average per-capita income with the national average. States with higher per-capita income averages are reimbursed by the federal government at a lower rate. Generally, FMAP cannot be less than 50 percent or more than 83 percent, according to federal law, although there have been some exceptions and temporary modifications.

The federal government funded 57 percent of total Medicaid spending in 2003, and states financed the balance. States are allowed to "impose nominal deductibles, coinsurance, or co-payments on some Medicaid beneficiaries for some services." However, cost sharing is not permitted for specific groups or services. In addition to matching state Medicaid spending on services provided to enrollees, the federal government matches state supplemental funding to hospitals that serve a disproportionate share of low-income patients.

What Medicaid services are provided?

States are given considerable flexibility in determining the scope of Medicaid services to be provided. However, federal law requires that certain services be provided if the state is to receive federal matching funds. These services include

- Inpatient and outpatient hospital services
- Physician, pediatric/family nurse practitioner, and/or nurse-midwife services
- Prenatal care
- Vaccines for children
- Early and periodic screening, diagnostic, and treatment services for children
- Family planning services and supplies
- Rural health clinic services and federally qualified health centers
- Laboratory and x-ray services
- Nursing facility services for persons aged 21 or older
- Home health care for persons eligible for skilled-nursing services

Designated optional services, such as diagnostic services, prescription drugs, prosthetic devices, or physical therapy services, may also qualify for matching federal funds if the service is provided by the state. Most optional Medicaid spending has been for long-term care and prescription drugs.[28]

What are the cost trends?

Federal and state spending on Medicaid was $266 billion in 2003, with 57 percent funded federally and 43 percent by states.

While the elderly and disabled represent only one-quarter of Medicaid enrollees, they accounted for 69 percent of Medicaid expenditures in 2003, with an average of over $12,000 per enrollee in this group. Medicaid spending averaged $1,700 per child and $1,900 for an adult using acute care services.

In 2003 over half of Medicaid spending was for acute care services, 36 percent was spent on long-term care services, and payments to disproportionate-share hospitals and for Medicare premiums accounted for the remaining costs.[29]

With double-digit cost increases and rising enrollment, Medicaid accounts for a growing share of tightening state budgets. States spent an average of 16.5 percent of their general funds on Medicaid in 2003, with some states spending nearly a quarter of their budgets on the program. Consequently, both the federal and state governments are looking at a variety of means to reduce costs, enrollment, and benefits.[30]

SCHIP and Other Government Programs

Congress created the State Children's Health Insurance Program (SCHIP) as part of the Balanced Budget Act of 1997. SCHIP expands health insurance coverage to children whose families earned too much to qualify for Medicaid but not enough to afford private insurance. Like Medicaid, SCHIP is a federal-state partnership. States have the option of using federal SCHIP funds to expand Medicaid coverage, to offer a separate children's health insurance program, or to create a combination Medicaid/SCHIP program. Federal funding for SCHIP programs is limited by law. For fiscal years 2005 and 2006, the federal contribution is set at just over $4 billion, and for fiscal year 2007 funding will increase to $5 billion. State allotments from the federal government are based on the number of children and a state cost factor.

Other public insurance programs include those provided by Department of Defense, the Department of Veterans Affairs, and the Public Health Service.[31]

Private Insurers and Managed Care

How did private insurance develop as the primary model for health care?

Private insurance funds most of the health care in the United States. According to the Census Bureau, just over two-thirds of Americans were covered by private insurance in 2003. Sixty percent were covered by employer-based group health insurance, while 9 percent purchased private insurance directly.[32]

Group health insurance grew out of the Great Depression in the 1930s, with the rise of Blue Cross programs offered by hospitals and, later, Blue Shield plans developed by physician groups. These local prepaid plans helped both providers and patients in a time of economic hardship. Blue Cross and Blue Shield plans evolved as not-for-profit organizations that were regulated by states differently than commercial insurers, and they captured a significant share of the health insurance market. The tax-exempt status of these plans was changed by Congress in 1986, and some Blue Cross Blue Shield plans have since converted to for-profit organizations.

With the advent of World War II, employer-sponsored health benefits became a popular means for recruiting workers in a tight labor market where wages were frozen by the government. Commercial insurers moved strongly into the health insurance market after the war. The private health insurance model in the United States was further strengthened when Congress opted not to tax employer contributions for health insurance as income for workers. These tax subsidies for employer-based health insurance currently cost the federal government over $100 billion a year in lost revenue. Concurrent attempts to establish a national health insurance program failed.[33]

What types of private group health plans are there?

Private group health insurance comes in a variety of forms. Most employers offer health benefit plans through a Blue Cross Blue Shield organization, through a commercial insurer, or through

self-insurance. In 2004 over half of covered workers were in a plan that was partially or completely employer self-insured, typically a preferred-provider organization.[34]

Traditionally, employers offered fee-for-service indemnity plans, in which the insurer reimburses the policyholder for the cost of care provided. In the late 1980s nearly three-quarters of covered workers were enrolled in fee-for-service indemnity plans; but by 2004, due to the expansion of managed care, nearly all covered workers were enrolled in some type of managed-care plan. Employees were most likely to be part of a preferred-provider organization (55 percent), a health maintenance organization (25 percent), or a point-of-service plan (15 percent).[35]

While managed-care plans played a role in slowing health care cost increases in the 1990s, they suffered a backlash from both patients and providers. As a result, some of their more restrictive characteristics have been eased or eliminated—in some cases by legislation.[36] Health care costs continue to rise, forcing some employers to discontinue health benefits. The percentage of Americans receiving health insurance through their employers decreased from 70 percent in 1987 to 63 percent in 2003, as shown in table 4–1.

How much does employer-sponsored health insurance cost?

Health insurance premiums have been rising sharply in recent years, increasing over 20 percent from 2002 to 2004. The employer-based health plan annual premium in 2004 was $3,695 for single coverage and $9,950 for family coverage. Employees typically contributed $558 (16 percent of the premium) for single and $2,661 (28 percent) for family coverage. Other employee cost sharing has become standard for employer health plans.

Table 4–1. Job-Based Health Coverage Is Declining

	Job-Based (%)	Purchased (%)	Public (%)	Uninsured (%)
1987	70.1	7.0	13.4	13.7
1990	67.8	6.8	14.6	14.9
1995	64.6	7.2	16.7	16.1
2000	67.1	6.6	14.1	16.1
2001	65.6	6.6	15.3	16.5
2002	64.2	6.7	15.9	17.3
2003	63.0	6.7	16.8	17.7

Source: P. Fronstin, "Sources of Health Insurance and Characteristics of the Uninsured," *EBRI Issue Briefs* (December 2003 and December 2004). Reprinted with permission.

Nearly all covered workers are responsible for co-payments or coinsurance for physician visits, while over half of workers now have separate cost sharing for hospitalization.[37]

What are consumer-directed health plans?

Consumer-directed health plans (CDHPs) are a new attempt to manage rising health care costs. Traditionally insured consumers often are insensitive to the costs of care and may even overutilize health services because their insurers, also known as third-party payors, have picked up the tab for their health care use. Getting consumers more involved in managing rising costs is the goal of CDHPs, primarily by shifting to them more financial risk and responsibility. This is done with high annual deductibles and greater co-payments or coinsurance. Although the particulars of CDHPs vary, consumers generally have more freedom to select their health care providers and medical benefits than is the case with other health plans. To help in decision making, most plans provide their members with prices and quality ratings for physicians and hospitals.[38]

To help ease cash flow in paying for these extra costs, CDHPs are usually coupled with a special tax-free savings account. Two types of accounts that have been created recently: the health reimbursement account (HRA) and the health savings account (HSA).

Health reimbursement accounts are funded and owned by the employer. Remaining account balances carry over annually but are lost when an employee leaves the company. HRAs are usually coupled with a high-deductible insurance plan, although that is not a requirement. In contrast, health savings accounts are employee-owned and must be combined with a high-deductible insurance plan. By law, the deductible must be at least $1,000 for single coverage and $2,000 for family. HSAs are portable across jobs, may be purchased by individuals, and may earn interest, and funds may be withdrawn and used for nonmedical purposes (subject to taxes and penalties for those under age 65).[39]

It's too soon to tell how effective consumer-directed health plans will be or what unintended consequences might arise. However, they are growing rapidly in the marketplace. HRA and HSA products accounted for 8 percent of insurer revenue in 2005, more than double that in 2004, and 72 percent of employers expect to offer employees an HRA or HSA in 2006.[40]

What are the trends in individually purchased health insurance?

Over 26 million Americans purchased health insurance directly in 2003. Purchasing health insurance as an individual is costly. There are greater administrative costs for selling policies one by one, and individuals must pay the full premium without an employer's subsidy. Individuals with preexisting medical conditions are at a disadvantage. They may have to pay more for coverage, coverage for the condition may be excluded, or coverage may be denied altogether. Some states have created high-risk pools or other methods to help, but success so far has been mixed.[41]

Age also affects the price of a policy. For a nonsmoking 25-year-old Chicago male, the average annual premium for an individual policy was $1,469 in 2005, but the premium for a 60-year-old male averaged $6,267.[42]

One recent study found that individually purchased health insurance plans also have higher deductibles and more meager benefits than group health plans. Individual insurance typically pays 63 percent of a health care bill, compared with the 75 percent that group health plans pay.[43]

For individuals who have lost their jobs, federal COBRA law guarantees them the right to purchase and continue their employer-based health coverage for up to 36 months. However, a former employee must pay the full cost of the premium plus an administrative fee of 2 percent. An individual could see the monthly premium rise from $42 for individual coverage as an employee to $288 for the same coverage as an ex-employee. For family coverage, the average cost could rise from $210 to $771 monthly, based on 2003 figures. Cost is a key reason that many decline COBRA coverage.[44]

How many Americans are uninsured?

Almost 45 million Americans—nearly one out of every six people—lacked health insurance coverage during 2003. The number has grown by 5 million a year since 2000. Surprisingly, 81 percent of the uninsured come from working families. Not all businesses provide health coverage, part-time or other workers may not qualify for benefits, and others cannot afford the premiums. Medicaid and other public insurance programs have limits in eligibility and benefits.[45]

With health benefit plans shifting more costs to the consumer, and in some cases restricting benefits, nearly 16 million adults under age 65 found themselves underinsured in 2003. The underinsured are those whose medical expenses totaled or exceeded 10 percent of their annual income (or 5 percent of income for those below the federal poverty level) or who had a health plan deductible equal to 5 percent or more of their income. The uninsured and underinsured accounted for over a third of the adult population under age 65 in 2003.[46]

Where do the uninsured get their care, and who pays?

Lack of insurance limits access to health care services. However, the uninsured still receive health care, paying for it out-of-pocket or shifting the cost to the health system. Nearly half of the uninsured may delay or forgo care, but deferred care can lead to more serious and costly medical problems. The uninsured are less likely to receive care, have poorer health status, and die younger than those with coverage. The uninsured accounted for nearly $99 billion of the nation's health care expenditures in 2001, and $35 billion of this was uncompensated care, not paid for by the individual or insurance. Uncompensated care costs are projected to rise to $43 billion during 2005.[47]

Hospitals, community health centers and other clinics, and physicians most often provide uncompensated care to those without insurance. The hospital share rose to nearly $25 billion in 2003. Community health centers and clinics provided over $7 billion in uncompensated care and physicians over $5 billion in 2001.[48]

Government and private sources underwrite some support for delivery of uncompensated care. For example, Medicare and Medicaid payments to disproportionate-share hospitals for their care of the indigent totaled about $8.4 billion in 2001. State and local tax appropriations support public hospitals and other facilities that provide safety-net care for the poor and uninsured. Tax exemption may be seen as another source of public support for private health care providers that must benefit their communities to maintain their not-for-profit status. Private charities play a role as well in delivering care to the poor. The cost of caring for the uninsured is reflected in the rising insurance premiums of those with coverage. According to one estimate, employer-based health insurance premiums were $341 higher for single coverage in 2005 due to the costs of uncompensated care. Uncompensated care has two economic components: charity care and bad debt. Charity care is provided without charge to the patient. Bad debt

results when patients or other payers default on charges.[49]

Ironically, the uninsured have sometimes been charged higher prices for health care, because they have not received the discounted rates negotiated by third-party insurers. Hospitals are doing more to make uninsured patients aware of their charity care policies or reduced-charge plans based on ability to pay. The challenge to health providers is to balance mission and margin, providing health care to those in need while maintaining financial viability.

Hospital Finances

Where does hospital money come from?

Most hospital revenue comes from third-party payors: Medicare, Medicaid, and private insurance. More than half of patient revenue now comes from government sources. The typical hospital gets 40 percent of its patient revenue from Medicare, 37 percent from private insurance, 13 percent from Medicaid, and the remainder from self-pay patients and other sources. While outpatient visits far exceed hospital admissions, inpatients still account for about two-thirds of patient revenue. Other sources, ranging from tax appropriations for government hospitals to cafeteria or gift shop sales, contribute other operating revenue. Investments and sales of assets contribute nonoperating revenue.[50]

Where does the hospital money go?

Labor costs account for more than half of hospital expenditures. Other costs are shown in figure 4–3.

The cost of hospital uncompensated care is usually reflected as a revenue loss rather than as a direct expense. However, charity care and bad debt account for about 6 percent of a hospital's costs. Federal laws, such as the Emergency Medical Treatment and Active Labor Act (EMTALA), guarantee patients hospital emergency care, but they do not guarantee funding for the care provided. Hospitals must absorb most of these costs.[51]

What are capital investment trends?

Hospitals must invest capital in their facilities, equipment, and medical and information technologies to maintain or upgrade these assets. From 1997 to 2001 capital spending by hospitals increased just 1 percent annually, not enough to keep up with depreciation rates. Capital spending is needed due to aging facilities, rising demand, changing technology, and marketplace pressure to stay competitive. Capital investment can lead to

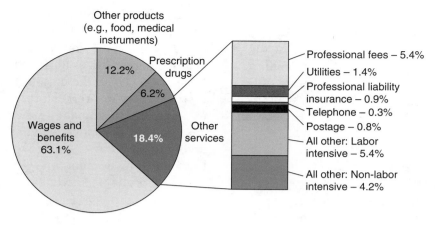

Other products (e.g., food, medical instruments) — 12.2%

Prescription drugs — 6.2%

Wages and benefits — 63.1%

Other services — 18.4%

Professional fees – 5.4%
Utilities – 1.4%
Professional liability insurance – 0.9%
Telephone – 0.3%
Postage – 0.8%
All other: Labor intensive – 5.4%
All other: Non-labor intensive – 4.2%

Does not include capital.

Source: Centers for Medicare and Medicaid Services, September 2004

Figure 4–3. Percentage of hospital expenditures (not including capital) by type, third quarter 2004.

Source: Lewin Group, *The Economic Contribution of Hospitals* (Chicago: American Hospital Association, February 2005), http://www.ahapolicyforum.org/ahapolicyforum/trendwatch/content/05econcontribwithtax.pdf (accessed June 22, 2005).

improvements in quality of care, patient safety, productivity, and staff recruitment and retention. However, the need for capital exceeds the supply, particularly with the fragile financial status of many hospitals. Total capital accessed by hospitals dropped from over $50 billion in 2001 to under $37 billion in 2002. The rate of and need for capital investment vary considerably among hospitals. However, in 2002 the median cost of hospital capital investment was about 7 percent of total operating expenses. Capital funding sources include tax-exempt bond issues, leasing, philanthropy, bank loans, and for-profit debt/equity. Capital investment will remain a significant challenge for the future.[52]

How are hospitals doing financially?

Many hospitals are struggling. Thirty percent of hospitals lost money in 2003, based on total margins, and 60 percent had negative patient margins. The difference between total margin, patient margin, and operating margin is defined in table 4–2. The majority of hospitals lose money treating Medicare and Medicaid patients. Medicare paid just 95 percent of hospital costs for the care provided Medicare patients, while Medicaid reimbursed only 92 percent. Since Medicare and Medicaid payments account for more than half of patient revenue in the average hospital, these government programs drive a facility's financial performance. Trends in hospital financial performance from 1990 to 2003 are depicted in figure 4–4.[53]

Government attempts to rein in the rising costs of the Medicare and Medicaid programs, in turn, shift costs to hospitals and other providers. To make up for the Medicare and Medicaid shortfalls, hospitals have shifted some costs to private insurers. Private insurance costs have been escalating, so businesses have shifted more costs to individuals. The number of uninsured increases, placing more stress on the system. And so the cost-shifting cycle continues. Most agree that these cost-shifting practices cannot be sustained in the long run.

What's the difference between hospital charges and hospital payments?

Hospitals establish chargemasters that list the fees for different services; however, the amount the hospital is *paid* for those services can vary. On average, Medicare pays only 43 percent of hospital charges, Medicaid pays 44 percent, and private insurance pays 52 percent.[54] In other words, more

Table 4–2. Types of Margins
• *Patient margin* indicates net income or loss based on patient revenues and expenses. Patient margins reflect a hospital's core business of caring for patients.
• *Operating margin* incorporates both patient and other operating revenues and expenses.
• *Total margin* includes net income from both operating and non-operating sources.

Source: J. Needleman, *Assessing the Financial Health of Hospitals* (Agency for Healthcare Research and Quality, December 2003), http://www.ahrq.gov/data/safetynet/needleman.htm (accessed June 27, 2005).

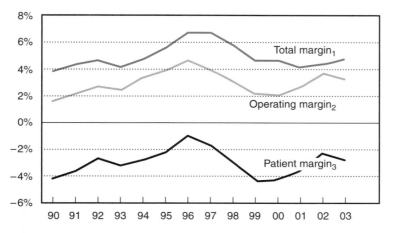

Source: The Lewin Group Analysis of the American Hospital Association Annual Survey data,1990–2003, for community hospitals

1. Total hospital margin is calculated as the difference between total net revenue and total expenses divided by total net revenue.
2. Operating margin is calculated as the difference between operating revenue and total expenses divided by operating revenue.
3. Patient margin is calculated as the difference between net patient revenue and total expenses divided by net patient revenue.

Figure 4–4. Aggregate total hospital margins, operating margins, and patient margins, 1990–2003.

Source: Lewin Group, "Trends in Hospital Financing," in *Trends Affecting Hospitals and Health Systems: TrendWatch Chartbook 2005* (Chicago: American Hospital Association, May 2005), http://www.ahapolicyforum.org/ahapolicyforum/trendwatch/ chartbook2005.html (accessed June 26, 2005).

than 90 percent of hospital patients pay less than the list price or charge for a hospital service. Like any business, hospitals establish their charges by forecasting their overall expenses and anticipated revenue.

What economic impact do hospitals have on their communities?

Hospitals employ nearly 5 million people nationally, ranking second only to restaurants as a source of private-sector jobs. Hospital jobs generally pay better than other service industry jobs and are more recession-proof. The purchase of goods and services by hospitals and their employees creates an economic ripple effect, adding over 7 million additional, related jobs to the economy. Nationwide, hospitals spent nearly a half trillion dollars in 2003.[55]

References

1. G. T. Savage, K. S. Campbell, C. D. Ford, and L. van der Reis, "International Health Care: A 12-Country Comparison," in L.F. Wolper, ed., *Health Care Administration* (Sudbury, MA: Jones and Bartlett, 2004); Organisation for Economic Co-operation and Development, "Private Health Insurance in OECD Countries" (Policy Brief, September 2004), http://www.oecd.org/dataoecd/42/6/33820355.pdf (accessed June 29, 2005).

2. Stephen Heffler, S. Smith, S. Keehan, C. Borger, M. K. Clemens, and C. Truffer, "U.S. Health Spending Projections for 2004–2014," *Health Affairs*, Web exclusive W5-75 (February 23, 2005), http://www.healthaffairs.org/ (accessed June 18, 2005).

3. Ibid.; Organisation for Economic Co-operation and Development, *OECD Health Data 2005: How Does the United States Compare?* (June 2005), http://www.oecd.org/dataoecd/15/23/34970246.pdf (accessed October 11, 2005).

4. U.S. Centers for Medicare & Medicaid Services, Office of the Actuary, National Health Statistics Group, "The Nation's Health Dollar: 2003" (January 11, 2005), http://www.cms.hhs.gov/ statistics/nhe/historical/chart.asp (accessed June 29, 2005).

5. U.S. Centers for Medicare & Medicaid Services, Office of the Actuary, National Health Statistics Group, "National Health Expenditures, Table 8: Other Personal Health Care Expenditures–Aggregate and Per Capita Amounts and Percent Distribution, by Source of Funds: Selected Calendar Years 1980–2003," http://www.cms.hhs.gov/statistics/ nhe/historical/t8.asp (accessed June 29, 2005); Craig Caplan and Normandy Brangan, "Out-of-Pocket Spending on Health Care by Medicare Beneficiaries Age 65 and Older in 2003," *AARP Public Policy Institute Data Digest* (September 2004), http://assets.aarp.org/rgcenter/health/ dd101_spending.pdf (accessed June 29, 2005).

6. Heffler, Smith, Keehan, Borger, Clemens, and Truffer, "U.S. Health Spending Projections."

7. BlueCross BlueShield Association, *Medical CostReference Guide* (Chicago: BlueCross BlueShield Association, October 2004), http://bcbshealthissues.com/issues/hccosts/pdf/mcrg_full.pdf (accessed June 29, 2005); PricewaterhouseCoopers, *Cost of Caring: Key Drivers of Growth in Spending on Hospital Care* (American Hospital Association and Federation of American Hospitals, February 19, 2003), http://www.aha.org/aha/press_room-info/content/PwCcostsReport.pdf (accessed June 29, 2005).

8. Elizabeth Docteur , Hannes Suppanz, and Jaejoon Woo, *The US Health System: An Assessment and Prospective Directions for Reform*, Economics Department Working Paper no. 350 (February 27, 2003), http://www.olis.oecd.org/olis/2003doc.nsf/43bb6130e5e86e5fc12569fa005d004c/a17bfa31f942be2cc1256cdb00332d3c/$FILE/JT00140050.PDF (accessed June 29, 2005).

9. U.S. Centers for Medicare & Medicaid Services, *Key Milestones in CMS Programs*, http://www.cms. hhs.gov/about/history/milestones.asp (accessed June 29, 2005).

10. Henry J. Kaiser Family Foundation, *Medicare at a Glance* (April 2005), http://www.kff.org/medicare/loader.cfm?url=/commonspot/security/getfile.cfm&PageID=52974&CFID=34174649&CFTOKEN=bbb2dbd34cf1425-915D29DB-054C-0ED4-D99628BC8E43BCE0 (accessed June 29, 2005); M. Nowicki, *The Financial Management of Hospitals and Healthcare Organizations* (Chicago: Health Administration Press, 1999).

11. Ibid.

12. U.S. Centers for Medicare & Medicaid Services, *Frequently Asked Questions*, http://questions.medicare.gov/cgi-bin/medicare.cfg/php/enduser/entry.php (accessed June 29, 2005).

13 .Henry J. Kaiser Family Foundation, *Medicare at a Glance*.

14. U.S. Centers for Medicare & Medicaid Services, *Frequently Asked Questions*.

15. Ibid.

16. Henry J. Kaiser Family Foundation, *Medicare at a Glance*.

17. Henry J. Kaiser Family Foundation, *Current Trends and Future Outlook for Retiree Health Benefits* (Menlo Park, CA: Henry J. Kaiser Family Foundation, December 2004), http://www.kff.org/medicare/7194/loader.cfm?url=/commonspot/security/getfile.cfm&PageID=49752 (accessed June 29, 2005).

18. U.S. Centers for Medicare & Medicaid Services, "Medigap Policy Basics: What Is a Medigap Policy?" http://www.medicare.gov/medigap/default.asp (accessed June 29, 2005).

19. Medicare Payment Advisory Commission, "Report to Congress: Medicare Payment Policy, Mar. 2005," http://www.medpac.gov/publications/congressional_reports/Mar05_EntireReport.pdf (accessed June 18, 2005).

20. Henry J. Kaiser Family Foundation, *Medicare at a Glance*; U.S. Centers for Medicare & Medicaid Services, *Medicare Administrative Expenses: Selected Fiscal Years* (November 2003), http://www.cms. hhs.gov/researchers/pubs/datacompendium/2003/03pg24.pdf (accessed June 29, 2005).

21. U.S. Centers for Medicare & Medicaid Services, *Background: Inpatient Psychiatric Facility PPS (IPFPPS)*, http://www.cms.hhs.gov/providers/ipfpps/ (accessed June 29, 2005).

22. U.S. Centers for Medicare & Medicaid Services, *Fact Sheet: Critical Access Hospital Program* (December 2004), http://www.cms.hhs.gov/medlearn/2CritAccssHospProfctsht.pdf (accessed June 29, 2005).

23. U.S. Centers for Medicare & Medicaid Services, *Acute Inpatient Prospective Payment System: Background* (September 16, 2004), http://www.cms. hhs. gov/providers/hipps/background.asp (accessed June 29, 2005); U.S. Centers for Medicare & Medicaid Services, *Acute Inpatient Prospective Payment System: Overview, Steps in Determining a PPS Payment* (September 16, 2004), http://www.cms.hhs.gov/providers/hipps/ippsover.asp (accessed June 29, 2005).

24. U.S. Centers for Medicare & Medicaid Services, *Definition and Uses of Health Insurance Prospective Payment System Codes (HIPPS Codes)* (May 28, 2003), http://www.cms.hhs.gov/providers/hippscodes/hippsuses.pdf (accessed June 29, 2005).

25. American Medical Association, *RBRVS: Resource-Based Relative Value Scale*, http://www.ama-assn.org/ama/pub/category/2292.html (accessed June 29, 2005).

26. U.S. Centers for Medicare & Medicaid Services, *Medicare Pay for Performance (P4P) Initiatives Fact Sheet* (January 31, 2005), http://www.cms.hhs.gov/media/press/release.asp?counter=1343 (accessed June 29, 2005).

27. U.S. Centers for Medicare & Medicaid Services, *Medicaid: A Brief Summary*, http://www.cms.hhs.gov/publications/overview-medicare-medicaid/default4.asp (accessed June 29, 2005); Kaiser Commission on Medicaid and the Uninsured, *The Medicaid Program at a Glance* (Henry J. Kaiser Family Foundation, January 2005), http://www.kff.org/medicaid/loader.cfm?url=/commonspot/security/getfile.cfm&PageID=50450 (accessed June 29, 2005).

28. U.S. Centers for Medicare & Medicaid Services, *Medicaid: A Brief Summary*.

29. Ibid.; Kaiser Commission on Medicaid and the Uninsured, *The Medicaid Program at a Glance*.

30. Henry J. Kaiser Family Foundation, *Distribution of State General Fund Expenditures, SFY2003*, http://www.statehealthfacts.org (accessed June 29, 2005).

31. U.S. Centers for Medicare & Medicaid Services, *Welcome to the State Children's Health Insurance*

Program, http://www.cms.hhs.gov/schip/about-SCHIP.asp (accessed June 29, 2005).

32. U.S. Census Bureau, "Income, Poverty, and Health Insurance Coverage in the United States: 2003, *Current Population Reports* P60, no. 226 (August 2004), http://www.census.gov/prod/2004pubs/p60-226.pdf (accessed June 29, 2005).

33. Rosemary A. Stevens, "Foreword," in Robert Cunningham III and Robert M. Cunningham, Jr., *The Blues: A History of the Blue Cross and Blue Shield System* (DeKalb: Northern Illinois University Press, 1997): viii; L.C. Gapenski, *Understanding Healthcare Financial Management* (Chicago: Health Administration Press, 2003); Alliance for Health Reform, *Covering Health Issues: A Sourcebook for Journalists* (Washington, DC: Alliance for Health Reform, 2004): 12, http://www.allhealth.org/sourcebook2004/toc.asp (accessed June 29, 2005); Claudia Williams, "Tax Subsidies for Private Health Insurance," in *The Synthesis Project* (Robert Wood Johnson Foundation, May 2003), http://www.rwjf.org/publications/synthesis/reports_and_briefs/pdf/no3_policyprimer.pdf (accessed June 29, 2005); S. Woolhandler and D.U. Himmelstein, "Paying for National Health Insurance: And Not Getting It," *Health Affairs* 21, no. 4 (July/August 2002): 88–98.

34. Gary Claxton, I. Gil, B. Finder, E. Holve, J. Gabel, J. Pickreign, H. Whitmore, S. Hawkins, and C. Fahlmann, *Employer Health Benefits: 2004 Annual Survey* (Menlo Park, CA: Henry J. Kaiser Family Foundation and Health Research and Educational Trust, 2004), http://www.kff.org/insurance/7148/loader.cfm?url=/commonspot/security/getfile.cfm&PageID=46288 (accessed June 29, 2005).

35. J. Gabel, G. Claxton, I. Gil, J. Pickreign, H. Whitmore, E. Holve, B. Finder, S. Hawkins, and D. Rowland, "Health Benefits in 2004: Four Years of Double-Digit Premium Increases Take Their Toll on Coverage, *Health Affairs* 23, no. 5 (September–October 2004): 200–209.

36. Docteur, Suppanz, and Woo, *U.S. Health System.*

37. Claxton et al., *Employer Health Benefits.*

38. Reden & Anders, Ltd., *Consumer Directed Insurance Products: Survey Results* (Chicago: American Hospital Association, April 2005), http://www.aha.org/aha/press_room-info/content/HSA.PPT (accessed June 29, 2005); Melinda B. Buntin, C. Damberg, A. Haviland, N. Lurie, K. Kapur, and M. S. Marquis, *Consumer-Driven Health Plans: Implications for Health Care Quality and Cost* (Oakland: California HealthCare Foundation, June 2005), http://www.chcf.org/documents/insurance/ConsumerDirHealthPlansQualityCost.pdf (accessed June 29, 2005).

39. Buntin et al., *Consumer-Driven Health Plans.*

40. Reden & Anders, Ltd., *Consumer Directed Insurance Products.*

41. U.S. Census Bureau, "Income, Poverty, and Health Insurance Coverage"; Alliance for Health Reform, *Covering Health Issues.*

42. Quotes obtained June 19, 2005, on www.ehealthinsurance.com, based on a Chicago location with a $1,000 deductible and 80/20 coinsurance.

43. Jon Gabel, K. Dhont, H. Whitmore, and J. Pickreign, "Individual Insurance: How Much Financial Protection Does It Provide?" *Health Affairs,* Web exclusive W172 (April 17, 2002), http://www.healthaffairs.org (accessed June 20, 2005).

44. Alliance for Health Reform, *Covering Health Issues.*

45. Catherine Hoffman, Alicia Carbauth, and Allison Cook, *Health Insurance Coverage in America: 2003 Data Update.* (Washington, DC: Kaiser Commission on Medicaid and the Uninsured, November 2004), http://www.kff.org/uninsured/loader.cfm?url=/commonspot/security/getfile.cfm&PageID=49550 (accessed June 29, 2005); Kaiser Commission on Medicaid and the Uninsured, *The Uninsured: A Primer* (Washington, DC: Kaiser Commission on Medicaid and the Uninsured, November 2004), http://www.kff.org/uninsured/loader.cfm?url=/commonspot/security/getfile.cfm&PageID=50811 (accessed June 29, 2005); Robert Wood Johnson Foundation, *About the Issue: Factsheets* (March 21, 2005), http://covertheuninsuredweek.org/factsheets/display.php?FactSheetID=101 (accessed June 29, 2005); Kaiser Commission on Medicaid and the Uninsured, *The Uninsured: A Primer.*

46. Cathy Schoen et al., "Insured But Not Protected: How Many Adults Are Underinsured? *Health Affairs,* Web exclusive W5-290 (June 14, 2005), http://www.healthaffairs.org (accessed June 29, 2005).

47. Kaiser Commission on Medicaid and the Uninsured, *The Uninsured and Their Access to Health Care* (November 2004), http://www.kff.org/uninsured/loader.cfm?url=/commonspot/security/getfile.cfm&PageID=49531 (accessed June 22, 2005); Kaiser Commission on Medicaid and the Uninsured, *Sicker and Poorer: The Consequences of Being Uninsured* (May 2002), http://www.kff.org/uninsured/20020510-index.cfm (accessed June 22, 2005); Jack Hadley and John Holahan, "How Much Medical Care Do the Uninsured Use, and Who Pays for It?" *Health Affairs,* Web exclusive W3-66 (February 12, 2003), http://www.healthaffairs.org (accessed June 22, 2005); Families USA, *Paying a Premium: The Added Cost of Care for the Uninsured* (June 2005), http://www.familiesusa.org/site/DocServer/Paying_a_Premium.pdf?docID=9241 (accessed June 22, 2005).

48. Hadley and Holahan, "How Much Medical Care Do the Uninsured Use?"

49. Families USA, *Paying a Premium*.

50. American Hospital Association, *Hospital Charges Explained* (December 2003), http://www.hospitalconnect.com/aha/key_issues/bcp/content/HospitalChargesExplained12803.pdf (accessed June 22, 2005); *AHA Hospital Statistics*, 2005 ed. (Chicago: Health Forum, 2004).

51. American Hospital Association, *Hospital Charges Explained*.

52. Healthcare Financial Management Association, *Financing the Future: Executive Summary* (June 2004), http://www.financingthefuture.org/400284a.ppt (accessed June 27, 2005); Solucient, *The Sourcebook: Comparative Performance of U.S. Hospitals* (Evanston, IL: Solucient, 2003).

53. American Hospital Association: *The Fragile State of Hospital Finances* (Chicago: American Hospital Association, 2005), http://www.aha.org/ahapolicyforum/resources/content/05fragilehosps.pdf (accessed June 22, 2005); *AHA Hospital Statistics*.

54. American Hospital Association, *Hospital Charges Explained*.

55. Ibid.; Lewin Group, "The Economic Contribution of Hospitals," *TrendWatch* 6, no. 1 (May 2004); *AHA Hospital Statistics*.

Chapter 5: Government and Other Types of Oversight

Jeanette M. Harlow

Each new regulation requires that a health care entity learn about the rule; conduct an analysis to determine how it changes current procedures; obtain approval for revised operating policies and systems; train staff; revise vendor contracts, if necessary; and establish methods for compliance documentation.

(American Hospital Association and PricewaterhouseCoopers, *Patients or Paperwork?* 2001)

Health care has often been described as one of the most regulated industries in the United States. Hospitals and other health care organizations face a complex array of federal, state, and local laws, regulations, and codes that affect all aspects of health care delivery. The variety of agencies that are involved in regulating hospitals at the state and federal levels alone is shown in figure 5–1.

Statutes and the regulations for implementing them may be ambiguous, contradictory, or subject to interpretation. In addition to the legal mandates that direct hospital activities, standards and guidelines developed by private organizations may give rise to a host of activities required to ensure compliance. Overlap among the various oversight agencies and organizations sometimes results in disjointed or duplicated efforts.

What is the impact on hospitals?

The sheer volume of regulations, advisories, alerts, rules, standards, and other guideline documents can be overwhelming. Medicare and Medicaid instructions alone have been estimated at more than 130,000 pages—about three times the size of the IRS Code and its related federal tax regulations. The amount of time, staff, and financial investment required to understand, implement, and ensure compliance with these requirements is enormous. A study conducted by PricewaterhouseCoopers on behalf of the American Hospital Association on the regulatory burden faced by hospitals found that paperwork added 30 to 60 minutes of work for every hour of patient care provided.[1]

Some of the activities a hospital must perform in order to implement a regulatory change are depicted in figure 5–2. The cost of health care regulation compared to its benefit in quality, economic, and social outcomes has been the subject of much debate through the years.

Noncompliance with regulations can incur stiff penalties for individuals or organizations. These may include fines, prison sentences, temporary suspension of payments, exclusion from participation in programs, or loss of tax-exempt status. The Department of Justice (DOJ) reported that in 2004, federal prosecutors filed a total of 395 criminal charges related to violations of health care statutes. In the same year, the federal government won or negotiated approximately $605 million in judgments and settlements in health care fraud matters. Additionally, 868 civil cases were filed, and 1,362 cases were pending. The Department of Health and Human Services (HHS) excluded 3,275 individuals and organizations from participating in the Medicare and Medicaid programs or other federally sponsored health care programs.[2]

A single hospital initiative may require scrutiny under multiple federal, state, and local laws and regulations. For example, a proposed hospital joint venture with another health care entity may involve issues related to antitrust, the anti-kickback law, physician self-referral prohibitions, or tax-exempt

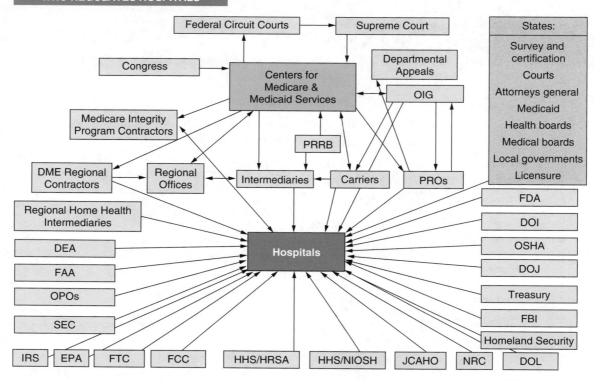

Figure 5–1. Government regulation of health care is cumbersome and confusing.

Source: American Hospital Association, *Overview of the U.S. Health Care System* (Chicago: American Hospital Association, February 2005), http://www.aha.org/aha/nhcp/content/Overview.ppt (accessed June 17, 2005).

status. Each of these potential impacts must be identified and addressed.

Health care organizations must ensure adherence to relevant regulations. An organizational compliance program can be a key tool in this effort. Under the U.S. Sentencing Guidelines for organizations, potential penalties may be significantly reduced by the existence of an effective compliance program and by proactive reporting, the assumption of responsibility, and cooperation with the authorities. The Office of Inspector General of the HHS has developed Compliance Program Guidance for Hospitals, which was originally published in 1998 and supplemented in 2005. These are voluntary guidelines to help health care organizations identify significant risk areas and evaluate and improve ongoing compliance efforts.[3]

Federal Government

The broad involvement of the federal government in health care is a relatively recent development in the United States. Until the twentieth century,

most governmental interaction with health care was conducted at the state and local levels. Key legislation contributing to the shift toward greater federal oversight will be reviewed in this section.

Role, Priorities, and Trends
What is the federal government's role in providing oversight?
The need to modernize hospitals following World War II led to the passage of the Hospital Survey and Construction Act of 1946, commonly known as the Hill-Burton Act. This act provided federal funds to the states to survey the need and plan for the construction of new hospitals. Projects that received funding through Hill-Burton had to comply with a number of requirements, including the provision of a level of charity care and community service. The Hill-Burton program was later expanded to include nursing homes and other facilities.

The National Health Planning and Resources Development Act of 1974 created federal, state, and local planning agencies that were involved in planning for new health care services, facility

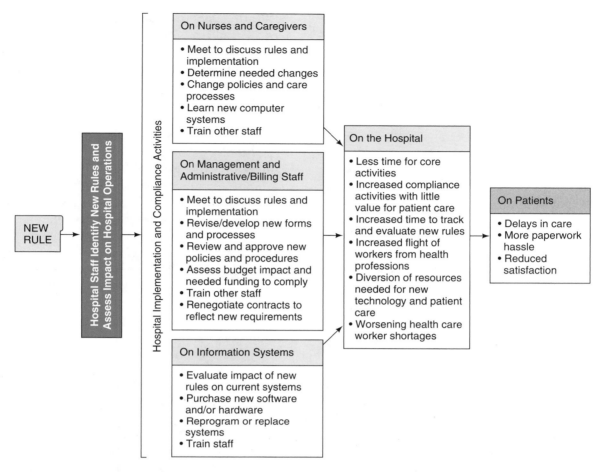

NEW RULE → Hospital Staff Identify New Rules and Assess Impact on Hospital Operations → Hospital Implementation and Compliance Activities

On Nurses and Caregivers
- Meet to discuss rules and implementation
- Determine needed changes
- Change policies and care processes
- Learn new computer systems
- Train other staff

On Management and Administrative/Billing Staff
- Meet to discuss rules and implementation
- Revise/develop new forms and processes
- Review and approve new policies and procedures
- Assess budget impact and needed funding to comply
- Train other staff
- Renegotiate contracts to reflect new requirements

On Information Systems
- Evaluate impact of new rules on current systems
- Purchase new software and/or hardware
- Reprogram or replace systems
- Train staff

On the Hospital
- Less time for core activities
- Increased compliance activities with little value for patient care
- Increased time to track and evaluate new rules
- Increased flight of workers from health professions
- Diversion of resources needed for new technology and patient care
- Worsening health care worker shortages

On Patients
- Delays in care
- More paperwork hassle
- Reduced satisfaction

Added government regulation imposes unfunded costs on hospitals.

Figure 5–2. One rule, many changes–many rules, countless changes.

Source: American Hospital Association and PricewaterhouseCoopers, *Patients or Paperwork? The Regulatory Burden Facing America's Hospitals* (Chicago: American Hospital Association, 2001): 6, http://www.aha.org/aha/advocacy-grassroots/advocacy/advocacy/content/FinalPaperworkReport.pdf (accessed June 21, 2005).

construction, and major capital expenditures, particularly for hospitals and nursing homes. The act introduced a regulatory approach to allocating health care resources and containing health costs. It also leveraged strong financial incentives to encourage states to adopt certificate-of-need (CON) programs, under which community need had to be documented, and within which certain new services and capital investment had to be approved. A network of health systems agencies at state and local levels administered the CON programs. Although federal statutory authority for the programs expired in the mid 1980s, many states have retained some level of CON regulation.

How has this role changed over time?
Federal involvement in the regulation of hospitals accelerated with the establishment of the Medicare program in 1966. As the role of government in funding health care has increased, so has regulatory scrutiny. In order to be eligible for reimbursement for care given to Medicare or Medicaid beneficiaries, hospitals must qualify as providers and meet the Medicare Conditions of Participation, along with other regulations that affect the programs. Because most hospitals are providers under one or both of the programs, these regulations have wide impact. In recent years, legislation such as the Stark Law has extended federal oversight beyond Medicare participating hospitals.

The Social Security Amendments of 1983 called for implementation of a Medicare prospective payment system (PPS) for reimbursement of most acute care hospitals. Under the statute, certain types of hospitals were exempt from PPS, including psychiatric, rehabilitation, long-term care, children's hospitals, and certain cancer hospitals.

The Balanced Budget Act of 1997 (BBA) made significant changes to the Medicare and Medicaid programs. It reduced Medicare spending, increased health care options for senior citizens by creating Medicare Part C (Medicare + Choice), improved Medicare preventive benefits, and gave states more flexibility in administering Medicaid. The BBA also created the State Children's Health Insurance Program (SCHIP) to expand health insurance coverage for children whose families do not qualify for Medicaid but who can't afford private insurance. As part of the statute, the Rural Hospital Flexibility Program created critical access hospital designations, allowing cost-based reimbursement for rural hospitals that meet defined criteria. The reimbursement systems for skilled nursing facilities, hospital outpatient services, inpatient medical rehabilitation, and home health services, which were previously exempt from the DRG (diagnosis-related groups, a list of categories used to classify treatment for reimbursement purposes) system, were to be converted from cost-based to prospective payment. Concerns over the financial impact of the BBA payment reductions led to the Balanced Budget Refinement Act (BBRA) in 1999 and the Benefits Improvement and Protection Act (BIPA) of 2000. The BBRA extended the prospective payment system to inpatient psychiatric services.

What are the key priorities today?

The federal government, in conjunction with state and local enforcement agencies, has placed an increased emphasis on controlling all aspects of fraud and abuse in the health care system, particularly Medicare and Medicaid. The most common types of fraud targeted include false claims, such as billing for services never provided; *unbundling*, or billing separately for services normally paid as part of a package; *upcoding*, or billing for a more complicated or expensive procedure than was actually provided; performing medically unnecessary procedures solely for the purpose of generating payments; or misrepresenting noncovered procedures as medically necessary in order to receive payments. Additionally, there is intense scrutiny of activities that violate laws related to referrals and compensation, mergers and acquisitions, and patient dumping.

The Health Insurance Portability and Accountability Act of 1996 (HIPAA) created a national Health Care Fraud and Abuse Control Program and established health care fraud as a federal criminal offense. In 2003, the Centers for Medicare & Medicaid Services (CMS) was allocated over $23 million to fund a variety of projects related to fraud, waste, and abuse in the Medicare and Medicaid programs, $10 million of which was specifically dedicated to combat fraud in the Medicaid program.[4]

What is the difference between a law and a regulation?

Statutes, or laws, are established by acts of legislature. A statute may be expressed in general terms, with the specific details delegated to the appropriate government agency to define and enact in regulations. Regulations are rules adopted by administrative agencies to implement, interpret, provide details, or govern the procedure of a law. Federal laws may also be interpreted through the judicial system, as individual court cases are heard and the bases for decisions are recorded in judicial opinions. These opinions have the force of law.

The first step in the legislative process is the introduction of a bill by a member of Congress. The bill is assigned a bill number that begins with "HR" in the House of Representatives and "S" in the Senate, and then it is referred to the appropriate committee or subcommittee that oversees the issues addressed in the bill. At this point, there may be committee or subcommittee hearings.

Key committees relating to health care issues in the House are Ways and Means, Energy and Commerce, and Education and Workforce. The House Ways and Means committee has jurisdiction over all of Social Security, welfare, and Medicare Part A, which pertains to hospital reimbursement. It shares jurisdiction with Energy and Commerce for other aspects of Medicare. Energy and Commerce has sole jurisdiction over the Medicaid program, and it oversees the Public Health Service. Education and Workforce relates to health care mainly through its oversight of the Employee Retirement Income Security Act (ERISA), which governs most employer-provided health insurance benefits. In the Senate, the Finance Committee oversees all of Medicare and Medicaid. The Health, Education, Labor, and Pensions Committee oversees public health services and has jurisdiction over ERISA.

Deletions or additions to the bill are made in "mark-up sessions," and the bill is reported back to the House or Senate, where it is placed on the calendar. Once the bill reaches the floor, substantial debate may ensue before a vote is taken. If passed, the bill is sent to the other house.

A bill must pass both the House and Senate before it is sent to the president for signature. If the House and Senate pass similar but different bills, members from each house form a conference committee to reconcile the differences. The conference report must be approved by both houses before the bill goes to the president. The bill becomes law when it is signed by the president or when his veto is overridden by both houses.

After legislation is signed into law, it may be referred to the appropriate regulatory agency for rulemaking. The way in which regulations are issued is generally directed by the requirements of the Administrative Procedures Act. Once the agency has analyzed the law's requirements, a proposed rule with the draft regulatory language is published in the *Federal Register* and made available for public comment for a period of time. The agency considers all the comments, makes revisions if needed, and then publishes the regulation again in the *Federal Register* as a final rule. The rule is then "codified" by being published in the *Code of Federal Regulations* (CFR), the official record of all regulations created by the federal government.

One of the most important annual pieces of legislation is the national budget, in which Congress defines federal revenue and spending targets for the fiscal year. The budget process is important not only because it sets funding for federal programs, but also because policy changes are sometimes added to appropriations bills. An outline of how the budget process works is shown in figure 5–3.

The budget process is kicked off each year in February, when the president sends his budget to Congress, identifying the administration's policy and funding priorities. By April 15, each house of Congress sets budget targets through a concurrent resolution that must pass both the House and the Senate in identical form. The budget resolution, which addresses the upcoming fiscal year and at least four succeeding years, establishes limits on discretionary spending for federal agencies and programs through spending allocations that are then divided into 13 suballocations, one for each of the appropriations subcommittees. The subcommittees draft the spending plans that are passed on to the full House or Senate Appropriations Committees, which may review and modify the bills and forward them to the floor for consideration. Once the House and Senate complete work on their respective appropriations bills, a conference committee is convened to iron out differences between the two versions. When the final bills are

approved in each chamber, they are sent to the president for signature.

Unlike the annual appropriations process for discretionary spending, mandatory spending, such as that for entitlement programs like Medicare, is typically provided for in the authorizing legislation and does not require annual action; however, mandatory spending must sometimes be adjusted to meet budget targets. In these cases, the budget resolution contains reconciliation instructions to the authorizing committees, resulting in reconciliation bills. Reconciliation bills have been a primary way that Congress has made changes—both fiscal and programmatic—to the Medicare and Medicaid programs.

Key Federal Departments and Agencies

What is HHS?

The Department of Health and Human Services (HHS), one of the largest federal agencies and the major federal regulator of hospitals, is charged with the mission of protecting the health of all Americans.[5] The Department of Health and Human Services carries out its activities through the following operating divisions: National Institutes of Health, Food and Drug Administration, Centers for Disease Control and Prevention, Indian Health Resources, Health Resources and Services Administration, Substance Abuse and Mental Health Services Administration, Agency for Healthcare Research and Quality, Centers for Medicare & Medicaid Services, Administration for Children and Families, and the Administration on Aging. The Department of Health and Human Services works closely with the Social Security Administration in the administration of the Medicare program.

The HHS Office of Inspector General investigates fraud and abuse in HHS programs, prosecutes civil monetary penalty and program exclusion actions, and makes recommendations regarding program improvements to prevent fraud and abuse. The agency also issues advisories, fraud alerts, bulletins, and other communications that clarify what is and is not permissible under existing statutes.

What is CMS?

Part of the HHS, the Centers for Medicare & Medicaid Services (CMS) administers the Medicare program and partners with the states to administer Medicaid and the State Children's Health Insurance Program (SCHIP). Health care organizations that receive Medicare reimbursement must meet the requirements stated in the

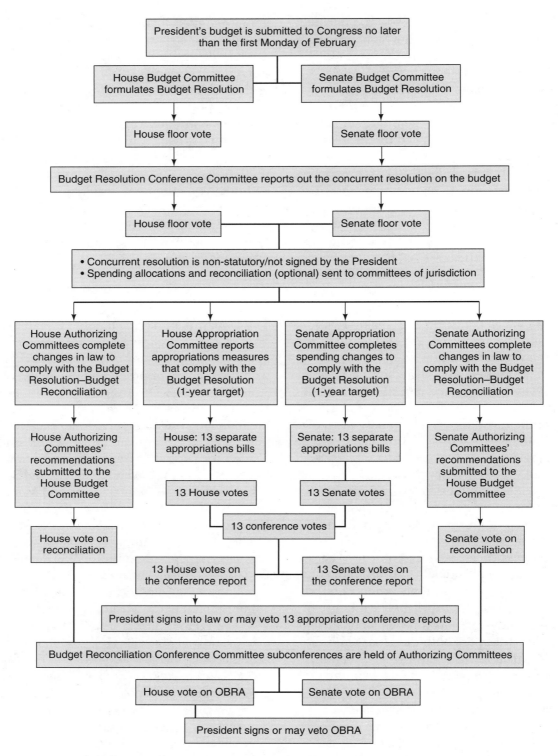

President's budget is submitted to Congress no later than the first Monday of February

House Budget Committee formulates Budget Resolution

Senate Budget Committee formulates Budget Resolution

House floor vote

Senate floor vote

Budget Resolution Conference Committee reports out the concurrent resolution on the budget

House floor vote

Senate floor vote

- Concurrent resolution is non-statutory/not signed by the President
- Spending allocations and reconciliation (optional) sent to committees of jurisdiction

House Authorizing Committees complete changes in law to comply with the Budget Resolution–Budget Reconciliation

House Appropriation Committee reports appropriations measures that comply with the Budget Resolution (1-year target)

Senate Appropriation Committee completes spending changes to comply with the Budget Resolution (1-year target)

Senate Authorizing Committees complete changes in law to comply with the Budget Resolution–Budget Reconciliation

House Authorizing Committees' recommendations submitted to the House Budget Committee

House: 13 separate appropriations bills

Senate: 13 separate appropriations bills

Senate Authorizing Committees' recommendations submitted to the House Budget Committee

13 House votes

13 Senate votes

House vote on reconciliation

13 conference votes

Senate vote on reconciliation

13 House votes on the conference report

13 Senate votes on the conference report

President signs into law or may veto 13 appropriation conference reports

Budget Reconciliation Conference Committee subconferences are held of Authorizing Committees

House vote on OBRA

Senate vote on OBRA

President signs or may veto OBRA

Provided by minority staff of the House Budget Committee, May 2004. For updates, go to www.allhealth.org

Figure 5–3. The budget process.

Source: Alliance for Health Reform, *Covering Health Issues: A Sourcebook for Journalists* (Washington, DC: Alliance for Health Reform, 2004): 142, http://www.allhealth.org/sourcebook2004/pdfs/appendixa.pdf (accessed June 21, 2005).

Conditions of Participation in the Medicare Program. The volume of regulations and instructions related to Medicare is extensive and is continually being updated through transmittals, memoranda, and other updates. The Centers for Medicare & Medicaid Services contracts with private companies, known as *fiscal intermediaries*, to process claims for Part A services (inpatient hospital care, skilled nursing facility care, home health care, hospice care, and hospital outpatient care). Coverage and payment decisions for Part B (physician) services are made by private insurance companies known as *carriers*.

What is the FTC?

The Federal Trade Commission (FTC), an independent agency that reports directly to Congress, enforces federal antitrust laws and works to prevent business practices that restrict competition, often in conjunction with the Department of Justice. The FTC investigates pricing strategies, mergers and acquisitions, and trends that have potential market impact, such as specialty hospitals.

What role does the EPA have in health care?

The Environmental Protection Agency (EPA) works to develop and enforce regulations that implement laws passed by Congress to protect the environment and the public from hazardous materials and pollutants. EPA standards address the management, storage, transportation, and disposal of wastes. Health facilities generate a variety of wastes from such diverse areas as administrative offices, housekeeping, laboratory services, surgical services, inpatient care, and clinical research. The types of wastes generated may include batteries, cleaning solutions, human pathological waste, municipal solid waste, biohazardous and infectious waste, pesticides, wastewater, air emissions, sharps waste, radioactive waste, mercury, and pharmaceuticals, to name a few. According to the EPA, there are more than 45 major federal regulations affecting air, water, and waste outputs from the health care industry.[6]

The EPA is responsible for researching and setting national standards for a variety of environmental programs, and delegates to states and Native American tribes the responsibility for issuing permits and for monitoring and enforcing compliance.

How does the IRS get involved with hospitals?

The Internal Revenue Service (IRS), a branch of the Treasury Department, administers the Internal Revenue Code and collects taxes for the U.S. government. For-profit hospitals are subject to the general tax rules that apply to other business organizations. Most hospitals in the United States, however, are not-for-profit entities, and these health care organizations interact with the IRS primarily on issues that impact their tax-exempt status. These issues include conflicts of interest, private inurement, executive compensation arrangements, financial incentives for physician recruitment, hospital joint ventures, unrelated business taxable income, and tax-exempt financing. Tax-exempt organizations with incomes of more than $25,000 must file IRS Form 990 annually to provide information on the organization's activities and finances.

Most not-for-profit hospitals are exempt from paying federal income tax as charitable organizations under section 501(c)(3) of the Internal Revenue Code and therefore must be operated to serve public rather than private interests. Although not explicitly defined, the provision of services that provide community benefit is a key factor considered when a facility's tax-exempt status is reviewed. Tax-exempt organizations must also meet requirements prohibiting private inurement of benefits, that is, using revenues for private, not charitable, purposes or providing benefit to an individual. Revenues derived from business that is not substantially related to the charitable purposes of the organization may be subject to unrelated business income tax (UBIT). Through the agency's Team Examination Program, large, complex not-for-profit health care organizations may be subjected to an intensive, line-by-line audit of their 990 forms. Recently, the IRS has identified the deterrence of abuse within the tax-exempt sector as one of its key objectives.

What role does OSHA have?

Due to the very nature of the work, there are a variety of occupational safety issues that arise in health care facilities. They can include biological hazards, such as needlestick injuries and other exposure to blood-borne pathogens; exposure to hazardous chemicals, drugs, gases, and other materials; exposure to tuberculosis and other infectious diseases; ergonomic stresses; and laser, x-ray, and radioactive materials hazards. The Occupational Safety and Health Administration (OSHA), established through the Occupational Safety and Health Act of 1970, develops and enforces regulations designed to protect health care workers from harm. OSHA is part of the Department of Labor.

How does the FDA relate to hospitals?

The Food and Drug Administration (FDA) is responsible for oversight of all medications and medical devices. As part of its mission, the FDA ensures the safety and effectiveness of drugs and vaccines, blood used for transfusions, medical devices, transplanted tissues, and equipment that uses radiant energy (such as x-ray machines). Health care organizations must track and report adverse drug reactions and problems with medical devices to the FDA.

Selected Laws That Affect Hospitals

Health Insurance Portability and Accountability Act

The Health Insurance Portability and Accountability Act (HIPAA, Public Law 104-91), enacted in 1996, includes provisions for significant privacy protections for personal health information. These provisions are far-reaching and impact the way this information is handled and by whom, how and where it is stored, what it is used for, and how and with whom it can be shared. Health care organizations must ensure not only that they comply with HIPAA privacy regulations, but also that affiliated entities and business associates who may have access to personal health information are in compliance. The administrative simplification requirements of the act seek to reduce the costs associated with many administrative and financial transactions by standardizing data and facilitating electronic transmission of health information. The act also includes provisions related to health care fraud enforcement, including the establishment of a program to coordinate the anti-fraud effort and a tracking system for the reporting and disclosure of adverse actions taken against providers, suppliers, or practitioners.

Emergency Medical Treatment and Active Labor Act

Part of the Consolidated Omnibus Budget Reconciliation Act of 1985 (COBRA), the Emergency Medical Treatment and Active Labor Act (EMTALA) is also referred to as the "anti-dumping" law. The statute requires hospitals to medically screen all patients who present themselves to the emergency department and to provide care to those with an emergency medical condition regardless of their ability to pay. EMTALA mandates apply to all hospitals that participate in the Medicare program.

Ethics in Patient Referrals Act

The physician self-referral statute was included in the Omnibus Budget Reconciliation Act of 1989 (OBRA 1989). Known commonly as *Stark I*, after Congressman Pete Stark, who introduced the statute, amendments to the legislation were included in the Omnibus Budget Reconciliation Act of 1993 (OBRA 1993) and became known as *Stark II*. Collectively, they are often referred to as the *Stark Law*. Under the Stark Law, physicians are banned from referring patients for designated health services to entities with which they or a member of their immediate family has a financial relationship. The relationship may be as an owner or investor in the entity, or it may be through a compensation arrangement. Stark II added to the list of designated services and extended the ban to Medicaid (Stark I applied only to Medicare-reimbursed services). Violations of Stark Law are civil in nature.

Antitrust laws

Antitrust activities have been addressed in a number of statutes, including the Sherman Act of 1890, the Clayton Act of 1914, the Federal Trade Commission Act of 1914, the Hart-Scott-Rodino Act of 1976, the Robinson-Patman Act of 1936, and succeeding amendments. Antitrust laws generally prohibit restraint of trade, creation of monopolies, and unfair methods of competition. In health care, areas of focus may include price fixing agreements, medical staff privileges, group purchasing arrangements, and mergers and acquisitions. Both the Federal Trade Commission and the Department of Justice Antitrust Division engage in enforcement activities related to antitrust. The Hart-Scott-Rodino Antitrust Improvements Act of 1976, which modified the Clayton Act, requires pre-merger review by the FTC and the Department of Justice for certain kinds of transactions.

False Claims Act

Originally passed into law in 1863 and amended in 1943 and 1986, the civil False Claims Act is a significant tool in combating fraud and abuse in government-funded programs such as Medicare. The act imposes substantial penalties for persons or entities who knowingly submit a fraudulent claim for payment to the U.S. government. An individual who knows of this activity (sometimes called a *whistleblower*) can bring a suit on behalf of the government and share in the money recovered. These suits, called *qui tam* suits, may be filed by employees, competitors, patients, or others.

Sarbanes-Oxley

The Public Company Accounting Reform and Investor Protection Act of 2002, more commonly known as the Sarbanes-Oxley Act, enacted sweeping reforms for the governance and accounting practices of publicly-traded corporations. Although not-for-profit organizations, such as hospitals and health systems, are not subject to Sarbanes-Oxley, they are likely to feel the effects of this legislation as its provisions become the standard for board accountability in both for-profit and not-for-profit organizations.

In a 2005 survey conducted by the Health Care Compliance Association, 74 percent of responders indicated that their organization had reviewed the Sarbanes-Oxley Act and determined that the following components applied to their operations:[7]

Conflict of interest	93%
Corporate responsibility for financial reports	73%
Code of ethics for senior financial officers	59%
Management assessments of internal controls	59%
Improper influence on conduct of auditors	47%
Disclosure of audit committee financial expertise	41%
Enhanced conflict of interest provisions	40%
Disclosures in periodic reports	32%
Public company audit committees	22%
Forfeiture of bonuses and profits	13%
Real-time issuer disclosures	12%

Medicare Prescription Drug, Improvement, and Modernization Act of 2003

The focus of this legislation, which is also known as the Medicare Modernization Act (MMA), is the provision of prescription drug benefits for senior citizens and disabled persons. The act also made provision for reimbursement to providers for emergency services furnished to illegal immigrants; enhanced reimbursement and expanded bed-size flexibility for critical-access hospitals; and continued funding of the Medicare Rural Hospital Flexibility Program grants. Included in the MMA was a temporary moratorium on physician referrals to specialty hospitals in which the physician has an ownership or investment interest, even if the specialty hospital is in a rural area.

Anti-Kickback Statute

The Medicare Anti-Kickback Statute (1972) makes it illegal to receive remuneration of any kind for referrals or services that are reimbursed under any federal or state health care program. Remuneration can include not only direct cash payments but also other types of incentives such as loan forgiveness, gifts, and discount leases. Certain "safe harbors" have been designated that define specific terms under which an arrangement will *not* be considered to be in violation of the statute. In order to violate the Anti-Kickback Statute, a provider or supplier must "knowingly and willfully" receive or pay prohibited remuneration. Violation of the statute may carry both criminal and civil penalties.

Civil Monetary Penalty Act

The Civil Monetary Penalties Act was passed in 1983 to prosecute fraud against federal health care programs such as Medicare and Medicaid and to assess monetary penalties against individuals, entities, agencies, or organizations. These penalties may be imposed in addition to penalties imposed by other laws.

Patient Self-Determination Act

Part of the Omnibus Budget Reconciliation Act of 1990, the Patient Self-Determination Act requires hospitals participating in Medicare or Medicaid to provide all patients with written information on policies related to self-determination and living wills. Health facilities are also required to determine whether patients have advance medical directives that define the conditions under which they might no longer wish to receive certain medical services.

Safe Medical Devices Act

The Safe Medical Devices Act of 1990 expanded the FDA's authority to regulate medical devices. The act requires hospitals and health professionals to report to the FDA if a device causes or contributes to patient injury, death, or other adverse experience.

Under the device tracking provisions of the act, hospitals are required to maintain records on patients who have received permanently implanted devices (such as pacemakers) and other life-sustaining devices used outside of hospitals (such as ventilators) so that these can be readily identified in the event that a potentially dangerous or defective device has to be recalled.

State Government

In the United States, regulation of health care traditionally has been focused at the state level; however, practices in the way states approach health care oversight vary greatly. These practices have developed over time and may have been affected by geography, demographic and cultural issues, financial resources, and the political climate. Even those areas of oversight common to all states, such as facility licensure, may differ considerably in scope and practice from state to state. It is essential that those responsible for making or overseeing decisions for health care entities be knowledgeable of state requirements related to their facility or type of organization. In some cases, business arrangements may cross state lines and require studying the laws of more than one state.

Role, Priorities, and Trends

As in the federal system, state legislatures enact statutes that govern activities within that state. State laws relate to federal laws in a variety of ways:

- State law may precede and form the basis of federal law.
- State laws may duplicate federal laws.
- State laws may duplicate federal laws in part but not in their entirety. (Except where specifically preempted by federal law, state statues must be followed. In some cases, there may be conflicts between the two sets of laws that must be resolved.)
- State laws may be preempted by, that is, superseded by, federal law.
- Federal law may provide a "floor" of requirements below which state law cannot fall.

Additionally, state administration, oversight, and enforcement of federally-funded or federally-mandated programs may be mandated by federal statute, as is the case with the Medicaid program.

Attorneys general are the chief legal officers of the states, and as such they have a primary role in issues related to antitrust prohibitions, environmental regulations, consumer protection, charitable trusts, Medicaid fraud, and other state-specific statutes and regulations. They may work in conjunction with their federal counterparts at agencies such as the Federal Trade Commission, the Department of Justice, the Environmental Protection Agency, and others.

Key Areas of State Oversight Activity

What is the state's role in Medicaid?

Medicaid is a jointly funded federal/state program that provides medical assistance for designated groups of individuals with low incomes or resources. Medicaid is administered at the state level by a single Medicaid agency in each state. Operating within broad federal guidelines, each state establishes its own eligibility standards; determines the type, amount, duration, and scope of services; sets the rate of payment for services; and administers its own program. As a result, Medicaid programs vary considerably from state to state. In order to receive federal matching funds, a state's Medicaid program must include certain basic services for designated populations. In addition to Medicaid, most states also operate "state only" programs that offer medical assistance to specified persons who do not quality for Medicaid.

To combat fraud and abuse in the system, states usually have Medicaid fraud control units, often located in the state attorney general's office, that pursue both criminal and civil actions against suspected providers. States have the right to impose civil monetary penalties, suspend payments, and suspend a provider from the Medicaid program; however, state actions must be in compliance with federal Medicaid laws and regulations.

What role does the state have in licensing?

States have always had the primary role in licensing health care providers. All states require that hospitals, nursing homes, and certain other health care facilities meet minimum standards of quality in order to receive and retain a license to operate. To receive Medicare or Medicaid reimbursement, health care facilities must be licensed under state law. State agencies (ordinarily the same ones who license facilities) are paid by CMS to survey facilities and determine whether they meet the requirements for Medicare certification. There is a set of specific requirements for each type of provider organization.

In recent years, with the increased emphasis on consumer empowerment and quality of care, some states have established programs to collect and publish data on hospital and nursing home costs or performance.

All states mandate licensure of physicians and certain other health care professionals. Licensure laws define minimum qualifications required to practice, as well as penalties for practicing without licensure and conditions under which licenses can be revoked.

Is certificate of need still around?

A certificate-of-need (CON) program establishes a process used by some states to control health care costs by regulating the proliferation of health care services, facilities, and technology. Hospitals operating in states with CON laws must obtain approval by a state health planning agency for capital expenditures related to major medical equipment, new construction or renovation, or the establishment of new services. In some states, hospitals are not subject to CON whereas other providers, such as nursing homes or ambulatory surgery centers, are regulated. In 2005, 37 states and the District of Columbia each had some type of CON program.[8] The efficacy of certificate-of-need programs in achieving their goals continues to be the subject of much debate.

What role do states play in rate review?

In reaction to the spiraling costs of health care in the 1970s and 1980s, some states developed hospital rate-setting programs that controlled prices hospitals could charge payors. These programs varied widely in terms of their voluntary or mandatory natures, the types of payors included in the program, and the ways in which rates were regulated. In addition to the cost-containment aspect, rate-setting systems could also incorporate allowances for uncompensated care into hospital rates, thus supporting access to care for medically indigent populations. With the rise of managed care and its potential for cost containment, states gradually abandoned these programs. Maryland is currently the only state that sets hospital rates.

What is the state's role in tax exemption?

Some states have enacted specific laws that exempt not-for-profit hospitals from state and local taxes, whereas other states have viewed the IRS criteria as the standard, and they generally accept federal tax exemption as adequate. At the state and local levels, health care organizations may be exempt from income, property, and sales taxes. They may also qualify under state law for tax-exempt bond financing—an important source of capital for not-for-profit organizations. States may require annual reporting for tax-exempt organizations, as does the federal government.

Under the state laws related to not-for-profit institutions, transactions that affect the assets of those institutions, such as merger with or conversion to a for-profit entity, may be subject to judicial review or approval by the state attorney general. In addition to issues related to the distribution of charitable funds, there may also be concerns about the impact of the conversion on the community's access to services. Assets are often transferred to a foundation charged with continuing to use the funds in ways that benefit the community.

The tax-exempt status of health care organizations has come under intense scrutiny in recent years. Not-for-profit hospitals and other health care entities face increasing pressure to justify their tax-exempt status at federal, state, and local levels. Some states have established explicit guidelines for the level of charity care or other community benefit that must be provided in order to maintain tax-exempt status.

How does the state regulate payors?

All states regulate the terms and conditions of health insurance sold in the state, including requirements related to health insurers' financial solvency. Most states mandate that insurance policies cover certain benefits, such as mammography screening or mental health services. Health insurers may be required to pay assessments, such as those for high-risk pools. High-risk pools provide health coverage for individuals who have been denied insurance coverage because of a medical condition.

Although they regulate health insurers, states are prohibited by the Employee Retirement Income Security Act (ERISA) from directly regulating employer-based health plans. Because self-funded health plans are not considered to be insurance, ERISA preempts them from state insurance regulation.

With the dramatic growth in managed care enrollment in the past decade, a growing number of states have passed legislation that addresses managed care plans. Many of these actions are focused on consumer protection, such as establishing ombudsman or consumer assistance programs; mandating consumer report cards that compare plans for quality, finances, and services; requiring specific sets or levels of benefits; or banning gag clauses that restrict a physician's ability to discuss all medically appropriate treatment options.

What other issues are covered by state laws and regulations?

Development of medical malpractice law has taken place primarily at the state level. The rules for handling malpractice cases have most often evolved as a result of decisions in state courts rather than through enacted statutes. As premiums for malpractice insurance have grown significantly over the last few years, concern over the malpractice claims system has also risen. Some states have enacted legislation known as *tort reform* to attempt to address the problems in the system.

Many states have adopted their own environmental regulations that are different from–and sometimes more stringent than–federal regulations. The EPA usually defers to or works cooperatively with state authority in enforcement actions. In 1999, a study by the Environmental Council of the States determined that 90 percent of all environmental enforcement actions were conducted by the states.[9]

Local Government

In the early days of this nation, a local government's role in health care was primarily related to its efforts to protect community health. These efforts later evolved into the creation of public health departments and, in some cases, public hospitals, such as county or city hospitals.

Role, Priorities, and Trends

States may confer specific powers to local governmental units, such as counties, towns, townships, municipalities, and districts. Local laws can never be weaker than federal or state law, and they are sometimes stricter. Local authority is typically limited to specific jurisdictional boundaries and cannot conflict with or impair federal or state law. Although city and county legislative bodies may adopt or adapt federal and state laws, there may be local variations. City or county authorities may have their own health facility licensure requirements, as well as related requirements such as parking regulations, building codes, waste handling requirements, and fire safety regulations. District attorneys and other local government prosecutors, such as city

attorneys, enforce state health care fraud and abuse laws.

What is the local role in tax exemption?

Because property taxes form the financial base of many local government services, the tax-exempt status of not-for-profit hospitals has become a controversial issue as municipalities face severe financial difficulties and look to hospitals as possible sources of tax income. Although hospitals' tax-exempt status has been traditionally viewed as being earned due to their community service commitment and relief of the government burden for care, some local governments have approached not-for-profit hospitals to request payments or contributions for local services in lieu of a formal tax assessment or municipal service charge.

Other Types of Oversight

As hospitals, other health care organizations, and health professionals seek to demonstrate their commitment to providing high-quality services, they may participate in a variety of activities related to accreditation and standardization.

Overview

What is accreditation?

Accreditation is the process by which an organization is recognized as meeting a set of predetermined standards. The development of standards for hospitals began in the early part of the 20th century when the American College of Surgeons (ACS) established five requirements as a minimum standard for hospital operations. The standards required hospitals to have an organized, competent, and ethical medical staff; rules, regulations, and policies to govern the work of the hospital; accurate and complete medical records for all patients; and adequate diagnostic and therapeutic facilities.[10] Today, accreditation is a highly complex and comprehensive activity. Accreditation organizations charge a fee for the survey and accreditation process, which must be repeated periodically.

Although accreditation is voluntary, it may also be used as an alternative to the Medicare survey and certification process. In order for an accreditation program to be used as the basis for Medicare participation, it must have been given "deemed status." Accreditation may cover most, but not, all Medicare requirements. Some states deem accredited hospitals to meet state licensure requirements.

Who establishes standards and guidelines?

In addition to the standards produced by accreditation organizations, standards may also be developed by professional or trade associations in the health care field. Standards may exist to ensure quality, increase productivity, or improve efficiency. They may address such diverse areas as technology, clinical practice, physical plant, patient care, medical devices, or professional development. The National Guideline Clearinghouse is a database of evidence-based clinical practice guidelines and related documents maintained by the Agency for Healthcare Research and Quality of the HHS.

What Are the Key Organizations?

Joint Commission on Accreditation of Healthcare Organizations

Created in 1951, the Joint Commission on Accreditation of Healthcare Organizations (JCAHO, or Joint Commission) is a private, not-for-profit organization that accredits the majority of U.S. community hospitals. Joint Commission accreditation has been deemed appropriate for participation in Medicare and Medicaid, so JCAHO-accredited hospitals are not required to undergo a separate survey process to participate in these programs.

The Joint Commission accredits hospitals, ambulatory care organizations, assisted living facilities, behavioral health care organizations, home care organizations, laboratories, long-term and subacute care organizations, managed care organizations, and office-based surgery programs. Because accreditation is not automatically renewed, a full accreditation survey is required at least every three years. The Joint Commission recently began using a new accreditation process in which all regular accreditation surveys will be conducted on an unannounced basis.

According to data from the American Hospital Association, 4,671 out of the 5,585 hospitals in the United States were accredited by the Joint Commission.[11] In recent years, a small number of hospitals have elected alternatives to Joint Commission accreditation, such as going directly to the state for their Medicare audits rather than using the "deemed status" conferred by Joint Commission accreditation; achieving ISO 9000 certification through the National Institute of Standards and Technology; or seeking accreditation through the

American Osteopathic Association's Health Facilities Accreditation Program (HFAP). A few hospitals maintain both Joint Commission *and* HFAP accreditation.

American Osteopathic Association

The American Osteopathic Association (AOA) implemented the Healthcare Facilities Accreditation Program in 1945 and accredits both allopathic (MD) and osteopathic (DO) facilities. The AOA program has been authorized by CMS to conduct accreditation surveys of acute care hospitals and hospital laboratories under Medicare. In 2005, there were approximately 136 HFAP-accredited hospitals.[12] The AOA has also developed accreditation requirements for ambulatory care/surgery, mental health, substance abuse, and physical rehabilitation facilities.

Commission on Accreditation of Rehabilitation Facilities

Established in 1966, the Commission on Accreditation of Rehabilitation Facilities (CARF) develops standards and accredits health care organizations for specific services such as adult day care, assisted living, behavioral health, medical rehabilitation, continuing care retirement communities and aging services, and child and youth services.

American Accreditation Healthcare Commission (URAC)

Originally established as the Utilization Review Accreditation Commission and now known simply as *URAC*, the organization also uses *American Accreditation Healthcare Commission* as a more descriptive corporate name. URAC maintains a wide range of accreditation programs, some of which address the entire organization and others that focus on a single functional area. Among the accreditation programs offered are case management, claims processing, health call centers, health plans, health websites, independent review, workers' compensation utilization management, credentials verification organizations, health care utilization management, HIPAA privacy and HIPAA security, and consumer directed health plans.

Accreditation Association for Ambulatory Health Care

The Accreditation Association for Ambulatory Health Care (AAAHC) was established in 1979 to develop standards for ambulatory health care organizations, including clinics, surgery centers, birthing centers, community health centers, diagnostic imaging centers, lithotripsy centers, managed care organizations, pain management centers, radiation oncology centers, urgent and immediate care centers, women's health centers, and others. AAAHC has been granted authority by CMS to certify ambulatory surgery centers for Medicare. A cooperative agreement with the JCAHO recognizes AAAHC accreditation as fulfilling JCAHO requirements for accreditation of ambulatory care organizations in certain situations.

National Committee for Quality Assurance

The National Committee for Quality Assurance (NCQA) began accrediting managed care organizations in 1991. Currently, NCQA has accreditation programs for a variety of organizations, including health maintenance organizations, preferred provider organizations, managed behavioral health care organizations, and disease management programs. NCQA accreditation is recognized by 30 states as satisfying certain regulatory requirements for health plans. NCQA also manages the Health Plan Employer Data and Information Set (HEDIS), a tool that measures the performance of managed health care plans. This data, along with NCQA accreditation information, forms the basis of a national database for health plan comparisons called Quality Compass.

National Fire Protection Association

The National Fire Protection Association (NFPA) establishes the codes and standards for fire prevention and safety that are referenced for the design and maintenance of health care facilities by state and local government agencies, the JCAHO, CMS, and other federal agencies.

American Institute of Architects

The American Institute of Architects (AIA), through its Academy of Architecture for Health and Facilities Guidelines Institute (FGI), publishes *Guidelines for Design and Construction of Hospital and Health Care Facilities*. The guidelines address minimum program, space, and equipment needs for various types of health care facilities, as well as engineering design criteria for plumbing, medical gas, electrical, heating, ventilating, and air-conditioning systems. The guidelines are used by most states and the JCAHO as a reference code or standard for licensure or accreditation.

American College of Surgeons

The Commission on Cancer (CoC), part of the American College of Surgeons, establishes standards for cancer care programs in hospitals, treatment centers, and other facilities. CoC-approved cancer programs are required to provide a defined set of basic services, either on-site, through referrals, or coordinated with other facilities or agencies.

References

1. American Hospital Association and PricewaterhouseCoopers, *Patients or Paperwork? The Regulatory Burden Facing America's Hospitals* (Chicago: American Hospital Association, 2001): 2, 12, http://www.aha.org/aha/advocacy-grassroots/advocacy/advocacy/content/FinalPaperworkReport.pdf (accessed June 21, 2005).
2. U.S. Department of Health and Human Services and U.S. Department of Justice, *Health Care Fraud and Abuse Control Program Annual Report for FY 2004* (September 2005), http://www.usdoj.gov/dag/pubdoc/hcfacreport2004.htm (accessed January 11, 2006).
3. Department of Health and Human Services, Office of Inspector General, "Publication of the OIG Compliance Program Guidance for Hospitals," *Federal Register* 63, no. 35 (February 23, 1998): 8987–8998; Department of Health and Human Services, Office of Inspector General, "OIG Supplemental Compliance Program Guidance for Hospitals," *Federal Register* 70, no. 19 (January 31, 2005): 4858–4876.
4. Department of Health and Human Services and Department of Justice, *Health Care Fraud Annual Report FY 2003*.
5. American Hospital Association, PricewaterhouseCoopers: *Patients or Paperwork?*
6. U.S. Environment Protection Agency, *Profile of the Healthcare Industry* (Washington, DC: Environmental Protection Agency, February 2005): 72, http://www.epa.gov/compliance/resources/publications/assistance/sectors/notebooks/health.pdf (accessed June 21, 2005).
7. Health Care Compliance Association, *7th Annual Survey: 2005 Profile of Health Care Compliance Officers* (Minneapolis, MN: Health Care Compliance Association, March 2005): 22, http://www.hcca-info.org/Content/NavigationMenu/ComplianceResources/Surveys/survey7.pdf (accessed January 11, 2006).
8. American Health Planning Association, *The CON Matrix of 2005 Relative Scope and Review Thresholds: CON Regulated Services by State* (Falls Church, VA:

American Health Planning Association, 2005), http://www.ahpanet.org/images/CONmatrix2005.pdf (accessed June 21, 2005).

9. R. Steven Brown and Valerie Green, *Report to Congress: State Environmental Agency Contributions to Enforcement and Compliance* (Washington, DC: Environmental Council of the States, 2001): 13, http://www.ecos.org/files/687_file_ECOS_20RTC_20f.pdf (accessed June 21, 2005).

10. *Manual of Hospital Standardization: A History, Development and Progress of Hospital Standardization: Detailed Explanation of the Minimum Requirements* (Chicago: American College of Surgeons, 1946): 6.

11. Don Nielsen and American Hospital Association, cited in "Hospital Oversight in Medicare: Accreditation and Deeming Authority," *NHPF Issue Brief* no. 802 (May 6, 2005): 9, http://www.nhpf.org/pdfs_ib/IB802_Accreditation_05-06-05.pdf (accessed June 21, 2005).

12. American Osteopathic Association, *HFAP Accredited Hospitals*, http://www.osteopathic.org/index.cfm?PageID=acc_hfhosp (accessed June 21, 2005).

Editor's note: Sources (in brackets) for the definitions are identified in the reference list following the final entry.

Academic medical center   Medical complex consisting of a medical school, university hospital, affiliated teaching hospitals, clinics, libraries, and administrative facilities **[AHA]**

Accreditation   Decision by an authorized credentialing body that an eligible institution or program meets applicable standards. A key accrediting body for health care providers is the Joint Commission on Accreditation of Healthcare Organizations. **[JCAHO]**

Acute long-term care   Specialized acute hospital care for medically complex, critically ill patients who have multisystem complications and/or failure and require hospitalization averaging 25 days **[AHA]**

ADC   (*see* Average daily census)

Admissions and discharges   Along with inpatient days, the most basic statistical measures of inpatient utilization. AHA asks hospitals to report admissions–the number of patients accepted for inpatient service, excluding newborns–during a given reporting period, usually a year. Other data collectors ask for a count of discharges–representing the completion of an inpatient stay. **[AHA, NCHS]**

Alliance   A formal organization that works on behalf of its individual members in the provision of services and products and in the promotion of activities and ventures **[AHA]**

ALOS   (*see* Average length of stay)

Alternative medicine   (*see* Complementary medicine)

Assisted living   A special combination of housing, supportive services, personalized assistance, and health care designed for those needing help in activities of daily living **[AHA]**

Average daily census (ADC)   The average number of inpatients on a single day during the reporting period, calculated by dividing the number of inpatient days by the number of days in the reporting period **[AHA]**

Average length of stay (ALOS or LOS)   A common benchmark of inpatient utilization referring to the average number of days that a patient stays at a facility. It is calculated by dividing the number of inpatient days by the number of admissions for a given period. **[AHA]**

Bad-debt expense   The provision for actual or expected uncollectibles resulting from the extension of credit **[AHA]**

Bassinets   Beds for babies, either normal newborns or those receiving special care in the neonatal intensive care unit **[AHA]**

Bed days   (*see* Inpatient days)

Bed size category   Grouping of hospitals based on the number of beds set up and staffed **[AHA]**

Beds, licensed   Number of beds authorized by the state licensing agency **[AHA]**

Beds, set up and staffed   Number of beds regularly available for inpatients, excluding bassinets and any beds for patients receiving special procedures for a portion of their stay who have other beds assigned to them **[AHA]**

Births   Number of babies born in the hospital, excluding fetal deaths **[AHA]**

Capitation   An at-risk payment agreement in which an organization receives a fixed, prearranged payment and in turn guarantees to deliver or arrange all medically necessary care required by enrollees in the plan

Census days   (*see* Inpatient days)

Center of excellence   A facility, department, or clinical service line with a reputation for superior quality of care; a designation often developed in competitive markets as a way to increase market share [Slee]

Certification Evaluation and recognition of an individual, program, or institution as meeting certain predetermined standards or requirements [JCAHO]

Charges Full established rates for services rendered [AHA]

Charity care Health services that were never expected to result in cash inflows, resulting from a provider's policy to furnish services free of charge to patients who meet certain financial criteria [AHA]

Community hospital (*see* Hospital, community)

Complementary medicine Organized services not based solely on traditional care as taught in most U.S. medical schools, including acupuncture, chiropractic, and herbal medicine, among others [AHA]

Control A type of organization responsible for establishing policy concerning the overall operation of hospitals. AHA has three main categories—government, nongovernment not-for-profit, and investor-owned—and numerous subcategories. [AHA]

Cost shifting The practice of increasing charges to a certain category of patients, such as private-pay patients, to make up for shortfalls in reimbursement from other payors [Slee]

Days, patient (*see* Inpatient days)

Deduction from revenue The difference between revenue at full established rates (gross) and the payment actually received from payors (net) [AHA]

Discharges (*see* Admissions and discharges)

Emergency department visits Number of visits to the emergency department, including those by patients who are later admitted to the hospital [AHA]

Expenses, total The sum of all payroll, non-payroll, bad-debt, and nonoperating expenses [AHA]

For-profit hospital (*see* Hospital, investor-owned)

Foundation A corporation, organized as a hospital affiliate or subsidiary, that purchases both tangible and intangible assets of one of more medical group practices. Physicians remain in a separate corporate entity but sign a professional services agreement with the foundation. [AHA]

Group practice without walls A quasi-group formed to share administrative expenses among physicians who otherwise remain independent practitioners [AHA]

Group purchasing organization (GPO) An organization whose primary function is to negotiate contracts for purchasing for members of the group or one that has a central supply site for members [AHA]

Health care system An arrangement usually comprising two or more hospitals that are owned, leased, sponsored, or contract-managed by a central organization [AHA]

Health maintenance organization (HMO) A managed-care organization that acts as both insurer and provider of specified health care services in return for prepaid payments [JCAHO]

Home health services The provision of nursing, therapy, and health-related homemaker or social services in the patient's home [AHA]

Hospice A program providing palliative care, primarily pain relief and supportive services, for terminally ill patients and their families, either in an inpatient setting or at home [AHA]

Hospital An organization or corporate entity licensed or registered by a state to provide diagnostic and therapeutic patient services for a variety of medical conditions, both surgical and nonsurgical [AHA]

Hospital, community Any nonfederal, short-term, general, or special hospital whose facilities and services are available to the public. Hospitals with nursing home units may be classified as community hospitals if the majority of patients are admitted to units with an average length of stay of

30 days or less. Community hospitals range from small critical-access hospitals to the largest academic medical centers, and may be not-for-profit or investor-owned. [AHA]

Hospital, critical-access   A small, rural hospital participating in the federal Critical Access Hospital Program, which was created in 1997 to improve Medicare reimbursement for limited-service hospitals by exempting them from the prospective payment system [Slee]

Hospital, general   A hospital that provides diagnostic and therapeutic services to patients for a variety of medical conditions, both surgical and nonsurgical [AHA]

Hospital, investor-owned   A hospital controlled on a for-profit basis by an individual, partnership, or profit-making corporation [AHA]

Hospital, long-term   A hospital with an average length of stay of 30 or more days [AHA]

Hospital, magnet   A hospital that has been recognized as demonstrating sustained excellence of nursing care [ANCC]

Hospital, niche   (*see* Limited service provider)

Hospital, primary care   A hospital offering basic services, such as emergency care, but limited intensive care or specialized services [DOJ]

Hospital, safety-net   A hospital that provides, through public mandate or its own mission commitment, a greater amount of care to the medically indigent [Slee]

Hospital, short-term   A hospital with an average length of stay of less than 30 days [AHA]

Hospital, special   A hospital that provides obstetrics and gynecology; eye, ear, nose, and throat; rehabilitation; orthopedic; and other individually designated specialty services [AHA]

Hospital, teaching   A hospital that has a medical school affiliation and offers training programs for medical residents, nursing students, or allied health students. The terms *major teaching hospital* and *university teaching hospital* are also used, typically referring to the flagship hospital in an academic medical center. [JCAHO, Slee]

Hospital, tertiary   A hospital that offers specialty and subspecialty services not found in primary care hospitals and that accepts referrals from other hospitals [JCAHO]

Indemnity fee-for-service   Traditional health insurance in which the insured is reimbursed for covered expenses regardless of the choice of provider [AHA]

Independent practice association   A legal entity that holds managed-care contracts and, in turn, contracts with physicians to provide care on a fee-for-service or capitated basis [AHA]

Inpatient days   The number of adult and pediatric days of care rendered during a reporting period (usually a year), excluding care for normal newborns [AHA]

Integrated delivery network   A local group that may include one or more hospitals, physician groups, outpatient facilities, health plans, or other community agencies working together to coordinate care [Slee]

Investor-owned hospital   (*see* Hospital, investor-owned)

JCAHO   (*see* Joint Commission on Accreditation of Healthcare Organizations)

Joint Commission on Accreditation of Healthcare Organizations (JCAHO)   Founded in 1951, the Joint Commission publishes standards, conducts on-site surveys, and accredits health care provider organizations in the United States. [JCAHO]

LOS   (*see* Average length of stay)

Licensed beds   (*see* Beds, licensed)

Licensure   Legal right to engage in certain professions or to operate certain types of facilities [JCAHO]

Limited service provider   A hospital or ambulatory care facility that focuses on a select group of services based on a clinical specialty (such as heart hospitals) or certain types of patients (surgical hospitals) [AHA-2]

Long-term hospital   (*see* Hospital, long-term)

Managed care   A broad spectrum of arrangements for health care delivery and financing, including health maintenance organizations, preferred provider organizations, point-of-service plans, direct contracting arrangements, and managed indemnity plans [AHA]

Network   A group of hospitals, physicians, other providers, insurers, and/or community agencies that work together to coordinate and deliver a broad spectrum of services to the community [AHA]

Occupied bed days   (*see* Inpatient days)

Outpatient visits   The number of visits by patients who are not lodged in the hospital while receiving services, including clinic visits, observation services, outpatient surgery, home health services, and emergency care [AHA]

Patient days   (*see* Inpatient days)

Physician hospital organization   A joint venture between a hospital and members of the medical staff in which they act as a unified agent in managed-care contracting, own a managed-care plan, provide administrative services, or own and operate clinical centers or services [AHA]

Point-of-service plan   A type of managed-care plan in which members are permitted to choose services either from a participating HMO or from an out-of-network provider. For out-of-network care, members must pay deductibles and a portion of the cost of care. [NCQA]

Preferred provider organization   A type of managed-care arrangement in which purchasers and providers agree to furnish specified health services to a group of employees/patients [AHA]

Prospective payment system   A reimbursement system, such as that used by Medicare, in which providers are paid predetermined rates for patient care services regardless of the actual costs of delivering that care [JCAHO]

Registered nurse   A nurse who has graduated from an approved school of nursing and is currently registered by the state [AHA]

Report card   A performance statement about a health care provider that is intended for use internally to improve operations, or externally as a means of comparison with other providers [JCAHO]

Revenue, gross patient   Revenue from all services rendered to patients at full established rates (charges) [AHA]

Revenue, net patient   Estimated net realizable amounts from patients, third-party payors, and others for services rendered [AHA]

Revenue, net total   Net patient revenue plus all other revenue [AHA]

Short-term hospital   (*see* Hospital, short-term)

Skilled nursing facility   An inpatient facility or unit that may be part of a hospital or nursing home in which medical, nursing, and other services are provided under the supervision of a registered nurse [AHA]

Special hospital   (*see* Hospital, special)

Swing beds   Hospital beds that can be used to provide either acute or long-term care depending on community or patient needs [AHA]

Trauma center   A facility that provides emergency and specialized intensive care to critically ill and injured patients [AHA]

Uncompensated care   Care for which no payment is expected or no charge is made; the sum of bad-debt and charity care absorbed by the organization in providing health care for patients who are uninsured or unable to pay [AHA]

Urgent-care center   A facility that provides care for walk-in patients with illnesses or injuries that are not true medical emergencies [JCAHO]

Visits, emergency   (*see* Emergency department visits)

Visits, outpatient   (*see* Outpatient visits)

References

[AHA]   *AHA Hospital Statistics*, 2005 ed. (Chicago: Health Forum, 2004).

[AHA-2]   *American Hospital Association, Protecting the Health Care Safety Net: Limited Service Hospitals* (Chicago: American Hospital Association, 2005), http://www.aha.org/aha/annual_meeting/content/05_limitedservhosp.pdf (accessed November 11, 2005).

[ANCC]   American Nurses Credentialing Center, *Magnet Recognition Program*, http://www.nursingworld.org/ancc/inside/about/aboutmagnet.html (accessed November 11, 2005).

[DOJ]   U.S. Department of Justice and U.S. Federal Trade Commission, "Chapter 3. Industry Snapshot: Hospitals," in *Improving Health Care: A Dose of Competition* (July 2004): 3, http://www.usdoj.gov/atr/public/health_care/204694.pdf.

[JCAHO]   Joint Commission on Accreditation of Healthcare Organizations, *Lexikon*, 2nd ed. (Oakbrook Terrace, IL: Joint Commission on Accreditation of Healthcare Organizations, 1998).

[NCQA]   National Committee on Quality Assurance, *A Glossary of Managed Care Terms*, http://www.ncqa.org/Programs/accreditation/mco/glossary.htm (accessed June 19, 2005).

[Slee]   Vergil N. Slee, Debora A. Slee, and H. Joachim Schmidt, *Slee's Health Care Terms*, 4th ed. (St. Paul, MN: Tringa Press, 2001).

Diversity, among health care professionals, 14, 17

Early diagnosis, role of, 7
Education. *See* Graduate medical education
Elderly population
    caregivers, role of, 28
    Medicare eligibility, 49
    poverty among, 2
    prescription drug coverage, 69
Electronic health records, 8
Emergency department use, 5–6
Emergency Medical Treatment and Active Labor Act (EMTALA), 55, 68
Employee Retirement Income Security Act (ERISA), 64, 71
Employer-based health plans, 53–54, 71
Environmental Protection Agency, regulatory role of, 67

False Claims Acts (1863, 1943, 1986), 68–69
Federal Medical Assistance Percentage, 51
Federal Register, 65
Federal Trade Commission Act (1914), 68
Federal Trade Commission, enforcement role of, 67
Fertility rate, 1
Financial performance of hospitals, 56
Food and Drug Administration, 68
    Safe Medical Devices Act (1990), 69–70

Gain sharing, between hospitals and medical staff, 20
Gastric bypass surgery, 6. *See also* Obesity
Genomics applications research, 7
Graduate medical education
    medical schools, 38
    payments for, 18
Group health insurance, 53–54

Hart-Scott-Rodino Act (1976), 68
Health Care Fraud and Abuse Control Program, 64
Health care reform, 5. *See also* Spending on health care
Health Facilities Accreditation Program, 73
Health insurance. *See also* Medicare program
    private insurance, 52–54
    State Children's Health Insurance Program (SCHIP), 52, 64
    state regulation of, 71–72
    uninsured population, 2, 51, 54–55
Health Insurance Portability and Accountability Act (HIPAA) (1996), 64, 68

Health reimbursement accounts, 54
Health savings accounts, 54
Health systems, 42–43
Hill-Burton Act. *See* Hospital Survey and Construction Act
Hippocratic oath, 1
Hispanics, in the health care workforce, 14
Hospitalists, 21
Hospitals. *See also* Children's teaching hospitals
    Certificate-of-need (CON) programs, 71
    clinical and administrative functions, 13
    community hospitals, 36–37, 38
    economic role of, 11–13
    finances of, 55–57
    growth in numbers of, 35
    in health systems, 42–43
    laws, effect of, 68–70
    limited-service, 20, 37–38
    magnet status, 23
    malpractice issues, 15
    Medicaid payments, 56–57
    Medicare payments, 50–51, 56–57
    physicians, relationships with, 19–20
    regulatory compliance, effect of, 61–62
    teaching hospitals, 18, 38
    utilization trends, 39
Hospital Survey and Construction Act, 35, 62
Human Cancer Genome Project, 7

Illegal immigrants, prescription drug coverage under Medicare, 69
Infant mortality rate, 3
Information technology in health care, 7–8
Inpatient care. *See also* Hospitals
    hospitalists, 21
    surgery, statistics, 6
Internal Revenue Service (IRS), 67
Invisible caregivers, 27–28

Joint Commission on Accreditation of Healthcare Organizations, 73

Licensed practical nurses, employment data, 12
Licensure, of health care professionals, 70–71
Limited-service hospitals, 20, 37–38
Long-term care, 41–42

Magnet hospitals, 23
Malpractice insurance, 15
Malpractice law, 72
Managed-care programs, 53
    accreditation of, 74
    state regulation of, 71–72